GROWING YOUNGER

RESTORE YOUR HORMONES, ENERGY AND SEX DRIVE

A POWERFUL NATURAL GUIDE TO OPTIMAL WELLNESS & LONGEVITY

GOWRI REDDY ROCCO, M.D.

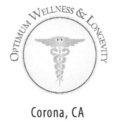

Corona, CA

GROWING YOUNGER
Restore Your Hormones, Energy and Sex Drive
A Powerful Natural Guide to Optimal Wellness & Longevity

ISBN: 978-1-7328598-0-7 (paperback)
ISBN: 978-1-7328598-2-1 (hardback)

Printed in the United States of America

Dedication

THIS BOOK IS DEDICATED TO MY LOVING FAMILY. TO MY wonderful husband, Robert, and my three amazing children, Robert, Jaya, and Nina. To my devoted mother, Jaya, and my father and role model, Dr. JMR Reddy; my loving brother, Viswa, and my beloved sister, Padma. My family is my inspiration, love and joy in life.

I am equally dedicating this book to all my patients over the years who have been my greatest teachers.

Disclaimer

THIS BOOK IS WRITTEN FOR EDUCATIONAL PURPOSES ONLY. This book is intended to supplement, not treat or diagnose any medical condition, and not to replace a patient/physician relationship. It is to offer alternative treatments and to educate based on the author's training, education, clinical experience, research and peer-review publications.

Please consult a health professional if you suspect you have a health problem or question. The author and publisher specifically disclaim any liability or loss through the use and application of any of the contents of this book.

Table of Contents

Acknowledgments

I WOULD LIKE TO THANK MY EDUCATORS, MENTORS AND professors throughout my academic and medical career. I have and will always remain a student. Thank you, AUC Medical School, for allowing me the opportunity to earn my Medical Doctor degree, even though I had to endure a volcano and hurricane to do so. Thank you to beloved, Dr. Kirk Hasanee, who was a monumental mentor in my career. He was the first to introduce me to Regenerative and Anti-Aging medicine, even before I completed my residency. I have been blessed to have worked alongside you. To Dr. Jeffery Levine, a mentor and my Women's Health Fellowship Director. He is a brilliant, gracious educator; he taught me to strive for excellence and balance being a doctor, wife and new mom, never to compromise family. I am grateful for his influence and demonstration of family, work and success. To Suzanne Somers, who has been a powerful advocate of bio-identical hormones and has been a great support and inspiration over the years. To Dr. Pamela Smith, my Anti-Aging Fellowship Director, thank you for inspiring me, teaching me, and keeping me a lifetime pupil.

Thank you, Norma Rede and Julianna Valtierra, for being wonderful staff and treating our patients with great care and love.

I would like to thank my lifelong friends, family and patients. Without all of you, I could not have written this book in its entirety. Thank you to my lifelong friends, Ajitha, Tiffany, Mala, Neha, Har and Raja. Thank you, Mayank Shah and your amazing team (Mai, Telma, Mike, Sam), Diane Ahn, Angela Haskins, Walker Evans, Sarah Palin, Dr. Alan Christianson and Dr. John West for your friendship and kindness. My loving friends, Angie L., Cathy E., Jenny E., Clare A., Janine H., Robyn D., Chris O., Janet W., Fatima G., Shelly S. and Lynn S. Thank you, Cassie, my spiritual sister and cousin.

I would like to thank my family, both my husband's and mine, who have all been God-sent. Amazing Powerful Love. Especially my husband's grandmother, Maria Caldarone, who's one of my favorite people in the world. She just turned 101 years old September 9. She's a strong, vibrant, beautiful woman. Thank you, Maria Rocco, my loving mother-in-law. Thank you to my precious parents. My mom, Jaya Reddy, fed us and any of our friends fresh, home-cooked food just about every night growing up, taught me grace, kindness and love, and exemplified how to be a great mother and homemaker. My father, Dr. Mohan Reddy, was the happiest hardworking person I've ever known, who taught me compassion, humility, tenacity and generosity. He smiles nonstop. He played Tony Robbins and Earl Nightingale on every road trip we ever took. He impassioned us to live with a purpose-driven life. Thank you to my sweet and wonderful brother, Dr. Viswa Reddy. He helps me see the truth and live in it. He is a stellar human being. My beloved sister, Padma Reddy, thank you. I serve, heal and help in honor of you. You inspire me daily, you were the most giving person I have ever known. My precious children, Robert Ram, Jaya Maria and Nina Lilly. My gifts from God. Thank you for giving me joy, laughter, hugs and kisses every day. My brilliant husband, Robert, thank you for your enduring love and support. You're a dedicated father, husband and doctor.

Finally, thank you to all my patients, my greatest teachers of all. Thank you for trusting me with your health and allowing me to help you to age healthier and grow younger!

Foreword

D R. GOWRI ROCCO IS ONE OF THE 'NEW KIND OF DOCTORS.' She has courageously stepped outside of the preset 'standard of care' box to offer information not learned in medical school. This new medicine takes into account the changing planet, the environmental assault and what we need to do to thrive and survive if we want to live a long and healthy life.

Dr. Rocco has a complete understanding of Bio-identical hormone replacement (BHRT), or, as I call it—'the game changer.' Hormones are the 'juice of youth' but, until recently, women and men were treated with a 'one-size-fits-all' patent medicine drug. No one was feeling well. True natural hormone replacement gives back quality of life and, in many cases, allows you to feel better than ever before in your life.

This is an informative, cutting-edge book that will educate you, allowing you to be in control of your health forever.

—Suzanne Somers

Iconic American actress, author, singer, entrepreneur, health advocate and spokesperson for bio-identical hormones.

A Whole Life Plan

Tell me and I will forget, teach me and I may remember,
involve me and I will learn.

— Benjamin Franklin

I HAVE BEEN COMPELLED TO WRITE THIS BOOK. I WANT TO provide a non-conventional pathway to aging better and living fully. Our healthcare system has failed us. It is like a GM assembly line, not custom-built. We must take accountability and seek out education for safe, do-able options to heal and age better.

People fear aging and all the usual symptoms that come with it: fatigue, insomnia, weight gain, brain fog, hair loss, depression, poor sex drive and life-threatening disease. Everyone knows someone close, or has personally endured cancer, diabetes, heart attack, obesity, stroke, Alzheimer's, high blood pressure or some other chronic disease. People are sick of taking tons of prescription medications every day without healing the disease or getting any better, but rather, sustaining the disease. Then, there are the side effects, which bring on a whole other set of medications to alleviate, just one after another.

The side effects of medications and the price of healthcare are astronomical. How do we feel better naturally? At every age, not just in our 20s?! How do we protect ourselves from these terrible medical conditions? How can we develop our own innate immune system to be so strong that it can combat existing disease, prevent new ones and live a long, healthy, youthful life?

In this age of massive information overload—internet, blogs, websites, I want to provide a simple yet powerful educational platform to transform your thoughts on disease and empower you to preserve your health and actually grow younger. I aim to provide a bird's eye view of health, looking at the forest, not the tree, kind of view. So many times, people focus on the minutia instead of the fundamentals of health. You have a *choice* every single day to engage in habits that grow disease and rob wellness or to engage in regenerating and preserving your stem cells and immune system.

People with multiple chronic illnesses and cancer often feel helpless and controlled by outside factors like medications and aggressive medical interventions. I will provide an intervention to existing illness to restore hope and help you gain control over your own health, so you can stop decaying and actually grow younger and healthier.

An important observation I made over my years of practice is that, generally, people tend to value money over their health. That is, until they lose their health. Then, they are willing to do whatever, and pay whatever, to fix their health. I remind my patients of what they already know—that good health is priceless.

I use the term "Bank your Health!"—just like people save money for retirement month-to-month and year-to-year, you should bank healthy habits day-to-day and month-to-month. It is important to understand that having daily, consistent healthy contributions to your "Health Savings Account" prevents disease, cancer and preserves long-term immunity and longevity! I will help you learn these healthy daily contributions to your health, so you can turn a state of helpless aging into a steady state of youthful agelessness.

I will introduce you to a powerful path to wellness and longevity. To heal and strengthen the immune system. A whole life plan! The topics I will discuss are all interconnected, a matrix of intentional wellness and earned health. You don't have to do everything or apply everything discussed. I am providing healthy options to give you choices. Do as many things as possible; balance and alternate them.

This book is my interpretation of health, gained over my 20 years of helping thousands of patients. I will share what I did to transform their health. There are three most valuable things in this world: Time, Health and Love. We cannot buy any of them. We must value each one of these and remember that without Health, we will be limited in our time with our loved ones. I am providing a platform of education and alternative options, so, as Jonathan Swift aptly put it, "May you Live ALL the days of your Life."

I esteem my relationship with my patients as a sacred partnership, based on trust and teamwork. I enthusiastically invite you to partner with me on this wellness journey, together; I will help you feel empowered to be healthier, live longer and feel younger.

Be excited, open-minded and proactive! These methods work for my patients and they will for you too!

Health and Happiness,

—GOWRI REDDY ROCCO, M.D., M.S.

PART I

Bio-Identical Hormones

CHAPTER 1

Optimizing Hormones Is the Secret to a Younger You!

You're never too old to become younger.

—Mae West

ACH ONE OF US IS UNIQUE. WE ARE A PRODUCT OF OUR GENES and our environment. This is what forms us and makes us unique from any other person. We are exposed to different stressors—toxins, diets, exercise, medications, trauma, sleep—and have different intrauterine birth experiences. We are born with a set of original genetic information called genes. So together, with your genes and your environment, "YOU" are formed. This is why we need to medically CUSTOM-treat and heal each person.

When we take a person's genetics and introduce health intervention, this actually alters their genes! This is called epigenetics. Epigenetics, as defined in the Merriam-Webster Dictionary, reads, "relating to, being, or involving a modification in gene expression that is independent of the DNA sequence of a gene." Basically, it means that even though type 2 diabetes may run in your genetic pool, you can prevent the expression of that gene in your life by improving how you eat, exercise, sleep, and balance your stress and hormones. Your epigenetic modifications can create a healthier, more disease-free YOU.

Surprising medical news has now reveled that our genetic makeup may not actually be a cause of many diseases, such as heart attacks, strokes, diabetes, obesity, dementia, etc., related with aging. In up to 75% of major life-threatening diseases, lifestyle and environment were the significant causes of onset of disease. The National Cancer Institute reported that only 5–10% of cancers are genetically inherited. The rest are determined by lifestyle and environment! How alarming and exciting! This means we play a huge role in how we age or don't age.

We have a CHOICE every day in how we choose to age. Daily thought and action determine how well and how long we live. We can age naturally or pathologically. Natural aging is wear and tear, accidents, and falls. Pathological aging means aging by disease and illness. I want to help teach you to age naturally and heal from pathological aging. Although I am traditionally trained as a medical doctor, I have continued my education and further trained as an anti-aging, functional and regenerative doctor. My focus is on prevention, a more natural disease intervention and healing process, to empower the body to heal itself. I have great respect for traditional Western medicine, and together with my training in alternative medicine, I feel armed with knowledge to use less medications and more lifestyle, nutritional and hormonal modifications to achieve optimal health and healing for my patients. It is important be open-minded and learn about progressive and natural options to live happier and age healthier.

Traditional medicine deals with treating the effects of aging. Anti-aging and Functional medicine deals with preventing the process of aging. The conventional belief is that as we age, our hormones decline. Rather, I subscribe to the neuroendocrine theory of aging: we age because our hormones decline. This is profound! We age because our hormones decline. Our hormones do not decline because we age.

This takes aging to whole other dimension of youth preservation and health empowerment! If we can restore and keep our hormones balanced, we can delay aging and its negative effects.

I will present to you a safe, natural way to restore your hormones, allowing you to transform your body back to health, improving your innate immune system, so you can feel energy, joy and vibrancy at any age. By restoring your hormones along with powerful lifestyle modifications, it is possible to actually grow younger! Let's begin with discussing hormones and why they are so important to our health.

CHAPTER 2

What Are Hormones?

*I have my hormones balanced. Most doctors are giving women
synthetic hormones, which just eliminate the symptoms, but it's
doing nothing to actually replace the hormones you have lost.
Without our hormones we die.*

—Suzanne Somers

HORMONES ARE BIOCHEMICAL MESSENGERS. THEY ARE chemical substances released from one part of the body that have an effect somewhere else in the body. There are messengers all over the body, giving and receiving signals. We have roughly 150 hormones. Most hormones are controlled by the hypothalamus, which sits in the brain. Hormones are produced by glands that are throughout the body. Hormones interact with each other, are "team players," are interdependent and need each other to keep the body optimally healthy. Some of the hormones are estrogen, testosterone, progesterone, DHEA, insulin, cortisol, TSH (thyroid stimulating hormone), HGH (human growth hormone), melatonin, and there are others.

Hormones tend to come in "a hormone pair," meaning one turns on and the other turns off. Hormones communicate organ-to-organ, tissue-to-tissue, and cell-to-cell. They turn cell functions on and off. They travel through the bloodstream to relay messages and determine everything from our immune system response, sexual development, metabolism, stress response, sleep, and how our body regenerates. Hormones are vital for repairing and regulating body functions. They incite, fortify and sustain cell healing and cell regeneration.

Hormones levels change throughout a lifetime. When hormone levels are at optimal levels and balanced, the result is a healthy body with a great immune system. Hormones have to be balanced as they are a complex network, and have opposing, synergistic, self-regulating feedback loops in place. We all have the same hormones. The ratios of sex hormones, estrogen to testosterone, determine female vs. male development. The right ratio, balance, and production of hormones are critical for feeling well. When aging causes a drop in hormone production, it causes a decline in the body's ability to repair and regulate itself.

Hormone levels are optimal and high for most people when they are 20 and 30 years old. Later in the mid- to late 30s, hormones start declining. During the 20 to 30 years that hormones are high and optimal, a person has energy, focus, is easily happy, sleeps optimally, has a strong immune system that wards off sickness, has less disease formation, has a strong sex drive, orgasms, loses weight easier, heals better, feels invincible and has great memory. From 35 years on, hormones steadily keep declining, with symptoms peaking around 40 and 50 years old. Declining sex hormone production in women is called menopause. Declining sex hormone production in men is called andropause.

As hormones decline, health declines: abdominal weight gain, low energy, poor sex drive, poor memory, headaches, poor attitude, poor sleep, onset of chronic diseases, feelings of weakness, poor healing, depression, anxiety, poor stress coping and feeling a victim to age. As hormones keep declining, there's a rise in obesity, type 2 diabetes, heart disease, cancer, dementia, strokes, autoimmune disease, sleep apnea and osteoporosis. Hormones decreasing dramatically increases the fat-to-muscle ratio to change.

Hormones are critical for cell growth and more importantly, cell repair, especially as we age. Low hormones prevent the immune system from repairing and regulating itself. Gene expression also gets altered by low hormones, meaning, too high or low of a certain hormone can express genetic disease or cancer. Hormonal decline varies person to person, depending on their genes and, more significantly, their lifestyle. Exercise, sleep, nutrition, the number and type of prescriptions they take and how they manage stress are all factors.

Restoring hormonal balance can prevent and treat the negative changes that can occur with aging. Restoring hormones regenerates our health; depleted hormones degenerates our health. The earlier you start restoring and balancing hormones, the healthier you age and the earlier you prevent disease formation.

Hormones can be restored safely and naturally. We will discuss the different hormones—sex hormones (estrogen, testosterone, progesterone, DHEA), thyroid hormones (TSH, T3, T4, reverse T3), stress hormones (cortisol) and metabolic hormones (insulin)—and how to safely and naturally restore and balance them using Bio-identical Hormone Replacement Therapy (BHRT). This is the first step in preventing premature aging, disease and death, along with healthy lifestyle modifications. With that said, BHRT isn't for everyone.

The rest of the book teaches you how to enhance your immune system, improve hormone production, with or without BHRT, increase lifespan, and prevent disease and cancer formation through powerful lifestyle modifications.

It is important to note that a hormonal imbalance can happen at any age, not just with menopause or andropause. Life is dynamic, and hormones are dynamic, changing with life situations. Here are several examples of hormonal imbalance related diseases: type 2 diabetes, thyroid disorders, PMS, postpartum depression,

PCOS (polycystic ovarian syndrome), obesity and depression. These hormonal imbalances can many times be fixed by diet modification, exercise implementation, and stress management, and vitamin supplementation, BHRT and natural thyroid medication, as needed. The following chapters will discuss this in detail.

HORMONES: ESTROGEN, TESTOSTERONE, PROGESTERONE, DHEA, THYROID, HGH AND CORTISOL

WHAT IS ESTROGEN?

Estrogen is a female sex hormone that is primarily made in the ovaries. Estrogen is the "primary" female hormone and a powerful "total" body hormone. Estrogen feminizes women and controls sexual development and female reproduction. There are estrogen receptor sites all over the body that require estrogen to function properly: uterus, bladder, heart, breast, brain, bones, liver, vagina, skin and blood vessels. These organs require adequate amounts of estrogen to properly function. I still remember my professor, Dr. Pamela Smith, lecturing, "Estrogen has over 400 critical functions in your body." Listed below are some significant ones.

WHAT ARE THE FUNCTIONS OF ESTROGEN?

- Maintains deep sleep
- Maintains sex drive
- Maintains vaginal moisture
- Maintains vaginal pH, preventing UTIs (urinary tract infections)
- Accelerates metabolism and fat-burning
- Increases energy
- Maintains fertility and pregnancy
- Maintains gut health by promoting good bacterial growth

- Increases serotonin in brain center to prevent depression & anxiety
- Decreases heart disease by 40–50%
- Decreases bad cholesterol, LDL and triglycerides
- Decreases arterial plaque
- Improves good cholesterol, HDL
- Reduces homocysteine, a cardiac and cancer risk marker
- Maintains blood vessel elasticity and increases blood flow
- Lowers platelet stickiness, which decreases risk of strokes and heart attacks
- Lowers blood pressure
- Decreases risk of colon cancer
- Has anti-oxidant properties, which improves immune response
- Regulates body temperature
- Prevents macular degeneration
- Prevents dry eyes
- Prevents tooth loss
- Helps with focus
- Maintains bone density
- Prevents and decreases wrinkles by making collagen
- Improves memory and cognition
- Improves mood by increasing serotonin levels

3 Major Types of Estrogens

There are three major types of estrogens: Estrone (E1), Estradiol (E2) and Estriol (E3).

Of the three, E2 is the most potent and biologically active hormone. E2 has anti-oxidative effects and reduces inflammation throughout the body organs. It is 12 times stronger than E1 and 80 times stronger than E3. It is responsible for most of the reproductive, cardiac, brain, bone, sleep, mood, and memory benefits. E2 is the main hormone produced from the ovaries up until menopause.

E1 is the dominant estrogen produced by the body after menopause. It is the "evil" estrogen. E1 prior to menopause is converted by the ovaries to E2. After the ovaries go into menopause, E1 doesn't get converted to safe estrogens. E1 is linked with breast and uterine cancer. In studies, alcohol has shown to increase E1 production, which in turn increases the risk of cancer. E1 is also produced from fat cells, the more body fat the more estrone produced. When E1 levels far exceed E2 levels, risk is higher for breast and uterine cancers. This is the connection between obesity, women, and increased cancer risks.

E3 is a weak estrogen, produced heavily during pregnancy, and it has been proven to have an anti-cancer effect. Research on mice showed that E3 may be able to prevent breast cancer. For these reasons, E2 and E3 are commonly used together for BHRT.

WHEN DO WOMEN START LOSING ESTROGEN?

Women start losing estrogen usually around 35 years old. By 40 years old, they lose about a third of estrogen and gradually keep losing estrogen until they hit menopause at about 50 years old, when they've lost up to 80% or more of their estrogen.

The hallmark of menopause is not having a period for one year. The ovaries stop producing estrogen. Perimenopause is the time from when estrogen slowly starts declining up until menopause when estrogen drastically drops. Perimenopause could last up to 10 years or more, ending in menopause. Menopause means the ovaries stop producing estrogen and progesterone, and a woman is no longer able to get pregnant. The average age of menopause in the US is 51 years old.

Perimenopause is a time of fluctuating hormones, with each woman feeling different symptoms, such as erratic periods, different from before, and usually heavier. Seventy to eighty percent of women get hot flashes, an overwhelming blast of heat that spreads to the whole body, causing agitation, difficulty focusing in daytime and preventing sleep at nighttime. Vaginal dryness is another symptom. Women lose vaginal lubrication and elasticity, and the vaginal wall become thinner, called vaginal atrophy. Sex becomes painful and not fun.

Women often get recurrent yeast and urinary tract infections. The vagina becomes more dry, itchy and irritated. This is very frustrating for women, especially when before they enjoyed their sex life, now they avoid it due to vaginal pain and dryness. It is also harder to climax and have mind-blowing orgasms. Stimulation takes a lot longer as well as time to climax, and often women become anorgasmic, meaning not able to achieve orgasms. The discomfort, lack of orgasm, and urinary tract infections (UTIs) deter women from trying. The vaginal dryness is frustrating for women, as their estrogen used to naturally lubricate the vagina, keeping it plump and thick, allowing painless and joyful sex. The hot flashes, along with the thinning vagina, itchy, recurrent yeast infections and UTIs, regardless of lotions and lubricants, makes life and sex frustrating.

Women also start gaining weight, especially in their abdominal region. Even with routine exercise and diet that worked before, they start gaining weight much more easily and find it harder to lose the weight. This is due to the drop in estrogen that burns fat and the rise in cortisol, the stress hormone that increases with age and causes weight gain. They start having mood swings, depression, anxiety, irritability and anger, and they find their moods fluctuate with their hormones. Less hormones, more mood swings. They feel a loss of control over their emotions. They also have a hard time falling asleep and getting back to sleep. They get night sweats and become insomniacs, waking up exhausted and feeling drained. This becomes a vicious, unhealthy cycle.

Some women enter into early menopause due to family history, smoking history, compulsive exercising, eating disorders, previous chemotherapy, history of long-term oral contraceptives, or due to surgical removal of the ovaries, uterine ablation, or surgical hysterectomy.

WHAT ARE SYMPTOMS OF LOW ESTROGEN?

- Hot flashes
- Night sweats
- Low sex drive
- Poor sleep, difficulty falling and staying asleep
- Insomnia
- Low energy
- Day-long fatigue
- Greater difficulty reaching orgasms
- Anorgasmic
- Painful sex
- Vaginal dryness, itching
- Vaginal odor
- Brain fog
- Poor memory and concentration
- Low energy
- Depression
- Anxiety, panic attacks
- Mood swings, irritability
- Poor confidence
- Loss of fullness in breast
- Headaches, migraines
- Facial hair
- Dry skin
- Dry hair
- Breakthrough bleeding
- Hair loss, shedding and thinning
- Weight gain, especially abdominal
- Wrinkles
- Sagging skin
- Joint pains
- Heart palpitations
- Frequent urinary tract infections
- Rise in bad and total cholesterol
- Rise in blood pressure, hypertension
- Rise in blood sugars, type 2 diabetes
- Muscle aches
- Food/carb cravings
- Difficulty losing weight
- Bloating, flatulence
- Acne
- Facial hair, especially chin and upper lip
- Itchy skin
- Dry eyes, skin and vagina
- Leaky bladder
- Osteoporosis/osteopenia
- Heartburn
- Dementia
- Heart attacks
- Strokes

After menopause, estrogen levels drop drastically. There are more than 45 million women in the U.S. going through either peri-menopause or menopause. Every year, about four million more women start with menopausal symptoms.

ESTROGEN AND HEART HEALTH

Scientific research shows a significant connection between menopause and heart disease. As soon as women hit menopause, their risk of heart attacks skyrockets, surpassing men. According to the Centers for Disease Control and Prevention (CDC), heart disease is the number one cause of female deaths in the U.S., killing almost 300,000 women in 2013. That's one in four female deaths (1 in 4!). That's more than twice as many deaths as all cancer deaths combined. Half of U.S. women don't even know that heart disease is the #1 female killer! What's worse, two-thirds of women who die suddenly of a heart attack have no previous symptoms. The biggest risk factors are high blood pressure, high LDL (bad cholesterol), and smoking.

After women start losing estrogen at about 35 to 40 years old, and a steeper decline after 45 to 50 years old, they easily gain abdominal weight, have an increase in bad cholesterol, have higher blood pressure and have a hard time burning sugar and fat, which can lead to insulin resistance and type 2 diabetes. They develop clogged arteries with a traffic jam full of sugar and cholesterol, which raises blood pressure, leading to heart attacks. Evidence shows that replacing estrogen with transdermal BHRT can reduce the onset of heart disease by 40 to 50%. This happens by lowering cholesterol levels, improving fat, sugar, and carbohydrate metabolism, and lowering blood pressure. In a large Finnish study where more than 7,944 women were followed for an average of seven years, the absolute risk for heart attacks was 50% lower in those women on estrogen replacement treatment.

Bio-identical estrogens have an antioxidant effect on free radicals and slow the development of heart disease by lowering bad cholesterol, LDL, raising good cholesterol, HDL, and reducing cardiac inflammatory markers. Bio-identical estrogens also have a vasodilatory effect on blood vessels, lowering vascular resistance and lowering blood pressure.

There is strong supporting evidence to start BHRT replacement as soon as low estrogen levels are detected in a woman and she's symptomatic. This helps to prevent risk of heart disease.

ESTROGEN AND BRAIN HEALTH

Estrogen helps maintain memory, improves thinking, improves mood, lowers depression, improves cognitive processing and protects neurons from decaying. It's reported that women are two to three (2–3) times more likely to get Alzheimer's disease than men. Although research is still being done on this topic, research has shown that estrogen protects brain cells from B-amyloid mediated toxicity (which is the cause of Alzheimer's disease) and from neuronal death in cell culture.

A study from Utah supports that women taking estrogen are protected from Alzheimer's disease and have a 40% reduced risk than their non-estrogen taking counterparts. The longer they remained on estrogen therapy, the lower their risk remained. Based on numerous other studies, long-term estrogen use prevents development of Alzheimer's disease in up to 60% of the female users.

REPLACING ESTROGEN PROTECTS AGAINST

Replacing estrogen protects against the following:

- Menopausal symptoms, especially hot flashes, insomnia, fatigue, vaginal dryness, weight gain
- Depression/anxiety
- Heart disease (decreases heart disease 40–50%)
- Stroke
- Alzheimer's disease
- Osteoporosis

WHAT IS TESTOSTERONE?

Testosterone is the "primary" male hormone and a powerful "total" body hormone. Testosterone masculinizes the man and controls sexual development and male reproduction. It is made primarily in the testes, and some in adrenal glands. Women also produce a small amount of testosterone in the ovaries. It is a total body hormone for men.

WHAT ARE THE FUNCTIONS OF TESTOSTERONE?

The main functions of testosterone include the following:

- Maintains sex drive
- Maintains erectile function and quality
- Maintains early morning erections
- Stimulates sperm production
- Promotes metabolism
- Sustains energy
- Burns fat
- Regulates blood sugar
- Builds muscle mass and strength
- Promotes immune system
- Lowers inflammation
- Lowers total cholesterol
- Maintains skin tone
- Promotes bone density
- Regulates prostate gland
- Mood enhancer
- Enhances mood
- Stimulates organ growth
- Promotes hair growth
- Provides feeling of assertiveness and decisiveness
- Provides confidence
- Improves cognitive function
- Improves memory
- Improves attention and focus

Testosterone peaks in men in their 20s and slowly starts declining in their mid- to late 30s. Total testosterone tends to be gradual, but free testosterone (the biologically active form) levels drop more drastically. Andropause, also called hypogonadism, is the male equivalent to female menopause. Andropause typically begins at 40 when the testes decrease testosterone production. After 30 years old, a man's bioavailable testosterone (the testosterone that is readily able to enter cells and be used by the body) level drops 2–3% annually.

Consequently, when bioavailable testosterone is measured in 50-year-old men, 50% of them are low in testosterone.

WHAT ARE THE SYMPTOMS OF LOW TESTOSTERONE?

The symptoms of low testosterone include the following:

- Decreased or absent sex drive
- Decrease in spontaneous early morning erections
- Decrease in erection fullness
- Decrease in ejaculation volume
- Decrease in sustaining erections
- Inability to achieve erections
- Decrease in orgasm quality
- Decrease in muscle mass
- Decrease in muscle endurance and strength
- Increase in body aches
- Increase in joint pain
- Muscle weakness
- Difficulty gaining muscle mass/tone/strength
- Fatigue, lack of energy
- Poor sleep
- Not dreaming
- Forgetfulness
- Loss of focus
- Lack of confidence
- Decreased work performance
- Decreased sports performance
- Lack of decisiveness
- Emotional, excessive fear and worrying
- Grumpy, irritable, mean
- Mood swings, negative thinking
- Depression
- Brain fog
- Decreased memory
- Decreased mental sharpness
- Decreased stamina
- Palpitations
- Easy weight gain, flabbiness
- Abdominal weight gain
- Dry skin
- Thin skin
- Breast formation
- Hot flashes
- Lost height, osteoporosis
- Rise in blood pressure or hypertension
- Rise in blood sugar or type 2 diabetes
- Rise in bad and total cholesterol
- Dementia
- Heart attack
- Stroke

Unlike women in menopause, men can naturally improve their production of testosterone with resistance training, weight loss, change in diet, and with more deep sleep. Most men, even with weight training and improved diet, still have low energy, poor sex drive, can't focus, have difficulty sleeping and a hard time losing weight. Free testosterone levels should be checked and bio-identical testosterone replacement therapy (TRT) should be started, especially if testosterone levels are suboptimal. Each man is unique, and treatment should be done on a custom basis. Bio-identical TRT is critical to preserve health and youthfulness.

A report published in the *Journal of Clinical Endocrinology and Metabolism* explains that since 1940, men of comparable ages are showing lower and lower levels of total testosterone. The researchers reported that testosterone levels have declined about 15% in men from 1987 to 2004. This may be due to lifestyle and environmental causes. Research shows that chronic stress, leading to high cortisol, is the major cause of low levels of testosterone in men.

A European study of more than 2,300 men showed the greatest longevity for men was with high testosterone. They reported a direct relationship of high serum testosterone and longer life. Another study of 11,606 men between the ages of 40 to 79 reported that men with high testosterone levels had lower mortality levels. They reported a 41% decrease of death when testosterone levels were greater than 564, compared to their counterparts whose testosterone levels were 350. For each increase in testosterone of 173 points, mortality rate dropped another 14%. They reported that with higher testosterone, there was no increase in prostate cancer and a lower death rate from heart disease. Most notable was that men with low testosterone had a high death rate from heart disease.

TESTOSTERONE AND HEART HEALTH

Numerous data show low testosterone in men is associated with increased risk of heart attacks, type 2 diabetes, and poor focus and memory. Low testosterone is associated with central obesity, increased systolic blood pressure and insulin resistance leading to type 2 diabetes. Testosterone replacement improves insulin sensitivity, so it helps fight diabetes and weight gain. Numerous studies have shown that low testosterone levels are associated with an increased risk for developing type 2 diabetes and metabolic syndrome (high LDL, low HDL, abdominal obesity, high blood pressure and insulin resistance). Metabolic syndrome is associated with an increase in heart disease, and an estimated 34% of the US adult population has this disorder. Due to this connection of low testosterone levels and increased risk of type 2 diabetes, the Endocrine Society recommends measuring testosterone levels in all men with type 2 diabetes.

Research shows that the heart muscle has more testosterone receptors than any other muscle in the whole body. Testosterone is critical for heart health. Men with coronary heart disease are low in testosterone. Testosterone lowers LDL cholesterol, the bad fat, and raises HDL cholesterol, the good fat. The higher testosterone and HDL levels, the more cardio protection a person has. There are many studies that show that higher levels of testosterone correlate with higher HDL, thus significantly reducing heart attack rates in men.

Testosterone replacement also reduces fat mass and increases lean muscle. The heart is the most important muscle, and restoring testosterone strengthens the heart muscle. Low testosterone is a common characteristic in men with heart failure; restoring testosterone has been shown to strengthen cardiac tissue, increase coronary blood flow and increase cardiac output. Testosterone also acts as a vasodilator, meaning it dilates arterial blood vessels and has shown to reduce angina.

World-renowned leading cardiologist and my one-time professor, Dr. Steven Sinatra, who wrote the book *The Sinatra Solution*, said that in order to treat and prevent heart disease, you need to consider BHRT along with CoQ10, L-carnitine and D-ribose.

TESTOSTERONE AND BRAIN HEALTH

Restoring testosterone increases blood flow to the brain. It restores memory and focus, improving mood and cognitive function. Testosterone has neuroprotective benefits. Several studies have linked low testosterone levels to increased risk of Alzheimer's disease in men. Testosterone replacement therapy (TRT) prevents formation of the Alzheimer's peptide, beta-amyloid precursor protein. Even in patients with Alzheimer's, the treated group improved over one year while the control group deteriorated. Testosterone also improves depression, restores energy, decreases abdominal obesity, builds bone and muscle strength and improves spontaneous erections.

Men start sleeping deeply again, wake up feeling more vital, have early morning erections again, start dreaming again and have a great sex drive with improved stamina and erection quality.

REPLACING TESTOSTERONE PROTECTS AGAINST

Replacing testosterone protects against the following:

- Andropause symptoms, especially fatigue, insomnia, weight gain and low sex drive
- Depression/anxiety
- Type 2 diabetes
- Heart disease
- Stroke
- Alzheimer's disease
- Osteoporosis
- Sarcopenia (muscle-wasting)

WHAT IS PROGESTERONE?

Progesterone is mostly a female sex hormone that balances estrogen, but it also is found in males in small amounts. It is made in the ovaries, adrenal glands and the placenta during pregnancy. It functions to maintain menstruation, pregnancy and sleep, down-regulates estrogen, promotes bone growth, protects against breast cancer, decreases fluid retention, protects brain cells, improves sex drive, lowers bad cholesterol, provides calmness and prevents anxiety.

During perimenopause, the ovaries pump out less progesterone. After menopause, progesterone levels drop drastically. Women can feel overly anxious, depressed, have poor sleep, and feel irritable, have horrible periods and headaches, and start gaining weight.

Restoring BHRT with progesterone helps balance estrogen and down-regulates estrogen receptors. It has an anti-inflammatory effect on the body and is neuroprotective and breast protective.

WHAT IS DHEA?

DHEA is a hormone secreted by the adrenal glands. It is a "prohor-mone," a precursor to both testosterone and estrogen. It also helps increase HGH (human growth hormone) levels in both sexes. It is an anabolic hormone with its highest levels during a person's 20s and diminishes with aging. DHEA is secreted at its highest levels between 4AM and 8AM. As cortisol levels rise from stress, DHEA levels decrease. Research supports that inflammation increases as DHEA decreases, and disease formation sets in with low DHEA levels. DHEA has protective effects, protecting a person from obesity, heart disease, cancer and autoimmune diseases.

WHAT IS HUMAN GROWTH HORMONE (HGH)?

HGH is the ultimate anti-aging hormone. It is called the "master hormone" because it affects every hormone and organ in the body to preserve youth. HGH, also called somatotropin, is made by the pituitary gland and released in bursts mostly during the "deep sleep" stage of sleep. It got its name from the fact that HGH release is necessary for children to grow in stature.

HGH regulates the body's metabolism of proteins, carbohydrates and fats, and helps to create lean body mass and strength. HGH also regenerates organs, increases energy levels, increases sex drive, strengthens the immune system, burns fat, improves mood, main-tains tight, firm skin, grows hair, keeps bones strong, helps lower cho-lesterol and blood pressure, and improves cognition.

IGF-1 is used as a clinical marker to determine HGH levels in the body. HGH levels drop like all the other hormones with age. IGF-1 levels start declining after the age of 25 and, by 40 years old, its levels fall by almost 50%.

Increasing HGH Can Be Achieved By

You can increase HGH by the following:

- Calorie restriction diet, reducing daily calorie intake by 10–20%, eating high-nutrient vegetables, fruits, proteins, low carb and sugars, and cutting out high-fat foods
- Healthy weight maintenance
- High intensity training or resistance training, 2 to 3 times a week
- Stress management
- BHRT hormone optimization
- Antioxidant supplementation, such as omega 3-fish oils, resveratrol, vitamin D3, and others listed later in this book
- Deep sleeping, 7 to 8 hours

WHAT ARE THYROID HORMONES?

The thyroid gland is the body's battery. It determines the body's metabolism, mood, energy, weight and blood circulation (which keeps the body warm.) The thyroid gland is shaped like a butterfly and sits at the base of the neck. The thyroid affects the entire body, and slight functional variations can have a dramatic impact.

Hypothyroidism, or low thyroid production, is commonly under-diagnosed and undertreated. All too often, patients come to get help because they feel horrible, but then they are told that their labs are normal and that there's "nothing wrong" with them. Patients feel tired, fat, can't focus, and feel depressed. They are told to just lose weight and work out. They're too tired and weak to do so! Why? Their thyroid is probably off!

Conventionally, the normal range for the thyroid is huge. TSH (thyroid stimulating hormone) is a parameter to check general thyroid function. The higher the TSH, the more hypothyroid or under-active it is. The conventional range is 0.2–5.0 mU/L. Who wants to be normal when today's normal is overweight, stressed out, tired, and hungry all the time? People need to feel extraordinary and well.

To achieve this, the optimum range for thyroid function should be 0.2–1.5 mU/L. Thyroid balance is critical to a person feeling energetic, positive, and ready to tackle the day—to losing weight, eating right and exercising.

What Are the Symptoms of Low Thyroid Levels?

Low thyroid levels are signaled by the following:

- Fatigue
- Cold hands
- Cold feet
- Constipation
- Dry skin
- Acne
- Hair loss and shedding
- Course, dry hair
- Brittle, weak nails
- Cold intolerance
- Poor sex drive
- Weight gain
- Increased appetite
- Headaches
- Slow speech
- Difficulty focusing
- Poor memory
- Dizziness/vertigo
- Decreased sweating
- Fluid retention
- Swollen ankles, feet
- Swollen eyelids
- Puffy face
- Depression, moodiness
- Nervousness
- Slow heart rate
- Heavy, clotting periods/painful periods/irregular periods
- Infertility
- Miscarriages
- Muscle and joint pain/weakness
- Morning stiffness
- Muscle cramps
- Horse, husky voice
- Excessive earwax
- Fibrocystic breasts
- Carpel tunnel syndrome
- High cholesterol
- High blood pressure
- Heart disease
- Obesity
- Insulin resistance
- Allergies, food and environmental sensitivities
- Eczema
- Loss of the last 1/3 of eyebrows
- Iron deficiency anemia

What Are the Symptoms of High Thyroid Levels?

High thyroid levels are indicated by:

- Fatigue
- Hair loss/shedding
- Excessive sweating
- Heat intolerance
- Goiter (enlarged thyroid gland)
- Weight loss
- Constipation
- Diarrhea
- Poor sleep
- Shortness of breath
- Chest pain
- Heart tremors
- Arrhythmias (irregular heart rate, usually racing)
- High blood pressure
- Tremors
- Light and irregular spread-out periods
- Nervousness, anxiousness
- Protruding eyes

Basic Thyroid Studies Needed for Thyroid Evaluation

The following are basic thyroid studies needed to evaluate your thyroid:

- TSH
- T3, total and free
- T4, total and free
- Reverse T3
- Thyroid antibodies: anti-thyroglobuin antibodies, anti-microsomal antibodies, anti-thyroperoxidase antibodies

Iodine deficiency is the most common cause, globally, for hypothyroidism. The most common cause of hypothyroidism in the industrialized world is auto-immune diseases. Iodine is essential for the thyroid to function properly. We don't make it and must get it from food sources or supplementation.

There are two main thyroid hormones, T4 (thyroxine) and T3 (tri-iodinethyronine). Both contain iodine molecules; T4 has 4 iodine molecules, and T3 has 3 iodine molecules. Without sufficient iodine, the thyroid gland cannot make adequate levels of thyroid hormones. According to my friend and colleague, Dr. Allan Christianson, and a leading expert in thyroid function, iodine deficiency may increase the incidence of thyroid autoimmune diseases; however, too much iodine intake can also contribute to thyroid imbalances. He reports too little or too much iodine is bad, and it needs to be just right. Too little iodine, less than 50 micrograms, can lead to iodine deficiency, goiter (thyroid enlargement) or hypothyroidism. Dr. Christianson recommends the right dose of iodine is usually between 100–300 micrograms a day and customizing on an individual basis is best.

The thyroid gland produces mostly T4. However, T4 has a minor role and must be converted to T3. When T4 loses an iodine molecule, it forms into T3. T3 is four to five times more potent than T4. Ninety percent of the thyroid receptors bind to T3. T3 is generally regarded as the biologically "active" hormone. T3 produces the desired thyroid effects: increased energy, metabolism and warmth. Conventionally, most patients with hypothyroidism are treated with medications for T4 only. Functional medicine doctors prefer treating it with a compounded thyroid replacement, using both T4 and T3. Compounded thyroid medication can be customized to each patient and their lab results with any specific ratio of T4 to T3. However, it is important to be monitored regularly.

One of the most common causes of hypothyroidism is Hashimoto's thyroiditis, an autoimmune disorder. This is when the body attacks itself and forms antibodies, which are detectable with blood testing. The antibodies listed above come back elevated on the blood work. Autoimmune disorders are 10 times more frequent in women.

T4 can also form rT3 (reverse T3). This is the inactive form of T3 and not desirable. The higher rT3, the lower the T3. Things that cause high rT3 are high stress levels, frequent weight fluctuations or yo-yo dieting, excessive alcohol, infections, aging, diabetes, prolonged illness, other hormonal imbalances, and environmental toxins. Things that can reduce rT3 are stress management, correcting an iodine deficiency, making sure ferritin levels and other hormones are optimal, detoxing with proper hydration, proper nutrition, regular exercise and supplements: B complex, vitamin D3, zinc, ashwagandha, fish oils, and vitamin C. These topics will be discussed in chapters to come.

Thyroid alone is not the "fix," It is part of the fix. Hormones, as discussed, are team players, they all work together. The sex hormones—estrogen, testosterone, progesterone and DHEA—have to work with the thyroid in harmony in order to feel well. Even if the TSH is in the optimal ranges, all other hormones have to be checked to assure proper hormone balance. The hormones are interactive, so one being off affects all the others. It's critical to check all hormones when evaluating a tired, overweight, depressed person.

Iodine

If you have a thyroid condition, iodine supplementation and dosing should be discussed, customized and monitored by your functional medicine doctor to prevent iodine-induced hyperthyroidism.

These are some brief properties of iodine:

- Antioxidant
- Anti-inflammatory
- Anti-bacterial and anti-viral
- Improves fibrocystic breast
- Necessary for optimal thyroid function

Foods rich in iodine—of all the foods, seaweed (kelp) is the most reliable source of natural iodine. Wild-caught seafood and fish, Himalayan or Celtic sea salt, cage-free eggs, organic, grass-fed meat and dairy, yogurt, beans, bananas, grass-fed butter, organic cheese, strawberries, green beans, and baked potatoes are also good sources of iodine.

Ferritin

Ferritin is a measure of iron stores necessary for oxygenation, energy and thyroid function. Hemoglobin, hematocrit and serum iron levels are often normal even if ferritin levels are low. In blood work, ferritin levels often drop before any of the other levels do. If ferritin levels are low, thyroid dysfunction commonly occurs. Ferritin levels could be low due to heavy periods, chronic blood loss or bowel disease.

Treatment of Low Thyroid

TSH levels are usually high and T3 is low. Functional doctors like to treat thyroid with customized dosing, just as they do with the other hormones. Conventional thyroid medications are pre-dosed and replace only T4. Customized or compounded thyroids replace both T4 and T3. The physician can customize the dose based on each patient and their lab results.

Treatment of High Thyroid

TSH levels are usually low, and T3 and T4 are high. The most common form of hyperthyroidism is Grave's disease, an autoimmune disorder. It is best to get a thyroid ultrasound and see an endocrinologist to rule out thyroid cancer or nodules.

WHAT IS CORTISOL?

As we age, all the hormones decline, except cortisol. Cortisol increases with aging and stress. It's infamously known as the "stress hormone." I call it the "evil" hormone, or the death hormone. In higher levels, it is a damaging hormone and counteracts all the other hormones. Cortisol is produced from the adrenal glands, a tiny lima-bean-size organ on top of each of our kidneys. When cortisol is balanced, it helps us manage the "fight or flight" events in our life, balances blood sugar and controls weight.

When we stress, we release cortisol, and when we relax, sleep, exercise, laugh, have orgasms, are enjoying life, and have balanced other hormones in our body, cortisol levels decline. The problem occurs when people stay in a state of chronic stress mode, exist in this mode and continue bad habits that keep them in this high stress mode. These bad habits include not exercising, eating processed foods full of bad fats and sugars, and drinking too much soda, coffee, energy drinks, and alcohol. They feel "burned out." High cortisol levels are responsible for annoying stomach fat, easy weight gain, stubborn weight that doesn't come off even with hard core exercise and proper eating, feeling depressed, poor sleep, overeating, gross daytime fatigue and nighttime alertness, restlessness and digestive problems.

Our hormones are like a seesaw with all hormones on one side and cortisol on the other. High cortisol negates all the other good hormonal effects in the body. With chronic stress and high cortisol levels are constantly released, your body produces more and more free radicals, which leads to inflammation, lowered immune system response and disease formation. Symptoms include increased stomach acid, headaches, brain fog, high blood pressure, poor sleep, sugar or salt cravings, bruising easily, heart palpitations, poor wound healing, mood swings, skin rashes, getting sick constantly, low sexual interest, high anxiety, exhaustion after exercising, excessive fat storage, and high blood sugars. Eventually the adrenal glands stop producing cortisol, and cortisol levels drop to low levels. Basically, the symptoms above just get worse and become your life, day in and day out. People feel exhausted, unwell and depleted. This is called "adrenal fatigue," a state of "burnout."

"Adrenal fatigue" was coined by one of my brilliant professors, Dr. James Wilson. His book *Adrenal Fatigue: The 21st Century Stress Syndrome* is a great book to read and explore this further. The best way to diagnose adrenal fatigue is to get a 4-point cortisol test by doing a saliva test, and/or to take Dr. Wilson's adrenal fatigue questionnaire. Most functional physicians are well versed on this topic and how to detect, test and treat it.

Adrenal fatigue can be treated. It is important to do so by evaluating all the hormone levels in the body, not just cortisol. When cortisol levels are too high, the body produces less progesterone. Progesterone and cortisol compete for similar receptor sites, and high levels of cortisol dominate the receptors. And, as discussed before, progesterone is the body's natural calming hormone for both men and women, helping in sleep, preventing anxiety and panic attacks, and improving mood. High cortisol levels also affect how the thyroid works. Remember the seesaw effect. It's important to check the levels of all hormones and delicately balance them. Hormones are team players and interconnected and, so, must work in harmony to feel good and function well.

Treatment is a customized hormonal balance and restoration, based on individual needs, followed with lifestyle and diet modifications. I discuss in following chapters the best power foods to eat and the proper lifestyle modifications to make regarding exercise, sleep, sex, detoxing, mental health and stress management. I detail high-quality supplements that help recover the immune system and regenerate stem cells after the chronic beat down of stress.

Most important is to avoid bad food choices, such as high caffeine drinks like soda and coffee. Have one cup of great tasting coffee in the morning. Avoid high sugar and fake sugars, and highly processed meats and carbs. Eat organic, plant-based foods and free-range meats only. Take a probiotic and drink decaf green tea, along with the supplements discussed later.

To reset cortisol levels, remove chronic stressors, get deep sleep, reintroduce a gentle workout plan like walking, have sex and orgasms every week, laugh, get "me" time and have your hormones—estrogen, testosterone, progesterone, HGH and thyroid—balanced. Happy, healthy bodies have balanced cortisol levels. The following chapters detail how to achieve this!

CHAPTER 3

What Causes Aging?

We don't stop playing because we grow old.
We grow old because we stop playing.

—George Bernard Shaw

THERE IS NO SINGLE THEORY THAT EXPLAINS WHAT CAUSES aging. Actually, scientists have postulated over 300 theories of aging. The causes of aging are all interlinked, and the most popular theory is actually the free radical theory of aging.

One theory of aging is that aging is caused by free radicals. Free radicals are different from other molecules in the body because they have a free electron, making them unstable molecules. This property allows it to react with other molecules in a highly volatile and destructive way. The free radical tries to get its missing electron filled by stealing it from molecules, near and far, impairing the cells along the way and creating extensive bodily damage.

Oxygen is the most frequent molecule to turn into a free radical. We breathe in oxygen all the time, so it's very available. These oxygen molecules can turn into free radicals (reactive oxygen species, or ROS) in the body by being damaged by too much sun exposure, high blood sugar, cigarette smoke, food and environmental toxins, prolonged levels of stress, sleep deprivation and overeating. Free radical damage over time causes age-related diseases like diabetes, heart disease, strokes, cataracts and cancer, and it can activate harmful genes.

Antioxidants are free radical scavengers. They are like "Pac-Man" eating up free radicals. When free radicals exceed antioxidants, the body is overwhelmed and oxidation stress happens. ROS causes a higher level of damage to cell membranes and cell mitochondria, and disturbs DNA and RNA synthesis, destroying and interfering with cell enzymes and protein synthesis, all of which causes low energy and fatigue, poor immunity and poor hormone function.

When oxidation stress occurs, we stop producing energy and feel tired all the time. More than 90% of the oxidation that occurs within living cells happens within the mitochondria. Mitochondria produce energy; they are the "powerhouse" in each of our cells. They are the engines of our cells. Mitochondria convert the fats and sugars we eat into chemical energy (ATP) using an oxygen molecule. Every cell of our body needs energy, in the form of ATP, to perform life-sustaining metabolic processes. Only mitochondria make ATP. Oxygen molecules, as discussed, can convert to free radicals. The more food we eat, the more oxygen that is required to make ATP.

Converting that to ATP is taxing on the mitochondria, so there is more potential for free radicals to be formed. This oxidative stress causes damage to the mitochondrial DNA, which can result in decreased ATP and energy production. This damage occurs throughout all tissues—heart, brain and skin, for example—and causes gross fatigue. It's been reported that by 80 years old, only about 4% of mitochondria are fully functional.

People eating excessive food, especially GMO (genetically modified organism, or genetically engineered) foods with toxins and pesticides that interfere with routine metabolism, can expect even more free radical formation and mitochondrial destruction. There-fore, scientists have concluded, eating less food in general means less free radicals in the body. It has been studied that 90% of free radicals in the body are the result of overeating!

This free radical formation and damage has been happening since birth and continues throughout our lifetime. When we are younger, the body can repair this damage more easily. As we age, repeated, accumulative effects of free-radical damage and oxidation stress have their effects, causing cell damage and mutations, ultimately leading to disease, cancer and death.

How Can We Decrease ROS Damage?

There are several ways to decrease ROS damage, including the fol-lowing. Eat less, manage and reduce prolonged stress, stop smoking, eliminate or reduce excessive sun exposure, eat whole organic, plant-based foods, and take antioxidants. Antioxidants, such as vitamins A, C and E, and beta-carotenes are monumental in destroying free radicals and stopping premature aging. Two of the strongest antiox-idants are polyphenols and flavonoids. We get these antioxidants through eating whole organic plant-based fruits and vegetables. Throughout this book, we will address these along with more pow-erful ways to decrease and prevent free-radical cell formation to stop premature aging and promote vital good health.

CHAPTER 4

What Are Bio-identical Hormones?

We age because our hormones decline.
Our hormones do not decline because we age.

—Neuroendocrine Theory of Aging

PEOPLE ARE LIVING MUCH LONGER NOW. ACCORDING TO THE CDC, the average life expectancy in the U.S. is 78.8 years. In 2017, life expectancy for men was 76 and 81 for women. The maximum lifespan of humans is about 120 years old. We have more centenarians now than ever before in time. We start declining in hormone production in our mid- to late 30s. That's living more than half our lives with barely any hormones! Remember, most of our sex hormones are depleted by the age of 50 to 55.

We need to preserve health, prevent disease and cancer for the second half of our life too, not to mention still have a great quality of life and maximum vitality! This is when most people think about retiring and traveling, enjoying the money they made—not exhausting their savings on health bills and drugs! The solution to preventing and treating symptoms of menopause, andropause, and age-related diseases is Bio-identical Hormone Replacement Therapy (BHRT) and lifestyle modification. The goal of BHRT is to safely achieve hormonal balance to more youthful levels to prevent premature aging, disease and cancer, and to regenerate stem cells to achieve longevity.

Bio-identical hormones have the same molecular structure as the hormones produced in the body. They are replicas of the body's own innate hormones. They are accepted, binding to the same receptors as the original hormone the body biologically produced, and are not seen as foreign chemicals. When they are not seen as foreign chemicals, the body incorporates the hormone and has minimal side effects. Bio-identical hormones are natural and made from plants (mostly wild yams, some come from soy) and have been used in medicine for over 50 years. Since bio-identical hormones are natural in origin, they cannot be patented, unlike their synthetic estrogen, progesterone or testosterone counterparts.

Bio-identical hormone replacement helps reset the body's hormonal clock to help delay the negative effects of aging. Each individual is unique and must be individually evaluated and custom-dosed. One size does not fit all. The right hormone balance helps manage and slow down aging. The wrong hormone balance accelerates aging. Customization is one of the best things about BHRT, making it safer for the patient and easier to titrate and monitor for the physician. Less is also more when it comes to BHRT, with routine follow-up visits and monitoring of hormone levels. The right hormone balance helps manage and slow down aging, treating the menopausal and andropausal symptoms, and mainly preventing heart disease up to 50%.

I will never forget one of my professors, Dr. Eric Braverman, saying, *"You're only as young as your oldest part."* So true! Implementing the right dose of BHRT is critical to restore and balance the entirety of the body systems to work in harmony again. With proper BHRT management, we can improve a person's physical and mental status by at least 10 to 20 years younger!

BHRT IS NOT FOR EVERYONE!

Bio-identical hormone supplementation is not for everyone. Each one of us ages differently; therefore, each person needs to be evaluated separately. After a one-on-one medical discussion, full evaluation, and review of hormone testing, a physician determines—along with labs and clinical symptoms—whether hormone imbalances and deficiencies exist; if so, BHRT is initiated.

If a woman or man is not a good candidate for BHRT and they don't have a true hormone deficiency or imbalance on lab studies, there are significant lifestyle changes that should be implemented to help them cope with symptoms. This is especially true for females having severe hot flashes.

It is most critical to fully evaluate thyroid function also. Many times, thyroid is overlooked by conventional medicine if TSH is in "normal" ranges. Detailed thyroid testing, including thyroid antibodies, as listed earlier, is critical for a deeper thyroid evaluation. This is especially true for a person who is overweight, obese or depressed, and has excessive hair shedding and dryness.

To get rid of menopausal or andropausal symptoms without BHRT, it is most critical to achieve a healthy weight, especially for an obese or overweight person. Avoid sugar, simple carbs, processed foods, dairy, caffeinated drinks, coffee, soda and alcohol. Eat abundant vegetables and organic whole produce, fish and meat. Eat more fiber-rich foods, such as lentils, beans, green leafy veggies, seeds, nuts, quinoa, fruit and root vegetables. Start a routine exercise regimen 4 to 5 times per week, at least 150 minutes a week. Research supports that regular exercise alone minimizes hot flashes, up to 55%. Resistance training is also important to build and maintain strong bones, preventing osteoporosis. Learn to manage chronic stress through healthy new habits, such as yoga, meditation, exercise, and deep breathing to avoid excessive cortisol production, the stress hormone responsible for weight gain, poor immune system response and poor sleep. Avoid tobacco and marijuana. Take medical-grade supplements (explained in the later chapter) to build up antioxidants, help empower the immune system and prevent disease. The rest of this book provides powerful tools to achieve all the above, with or without BHRT implementation.

Just implementing the compelling lifestyle changes in this book will transform your body into a younger, vibrant, healthier state of well-being and extend your lifespan.

BHRT IMPLEMENTATION

Clinical signs and symptoms are primary in hormonal evaluations. In anti-aging medicine, we do not "treat by numbers" only. It is critical to assess the person as a whole to determine quality of life, evaluate lab results, and safely initiate BHRT. Prescribing BHRT requires specialized training, so it is critical to seek out a highly qualified, well-trained physician. Dosing is low and slow. Delivering safe, routinely regulated, physiologically optimal levels is key. The balance of hormones is more important than the actual levels. In women, ratios of estrogen to progesterone and estrogen to testosterone are important. And in men, the ratio of testosterone to estrogen is important.

I recommend transdermal BHRT, low-dosed rub-on creams, customized and prescribed by a physician, made by a PCAB-accredited compounding pharmacy, precisely calibrated in applicators, and applied to the inner thigh, buttock or love handles area. The goal is to reach physiological levels with the lowest doses possible to support cardiac, brain, bone, sleep, and metabolic health and alleviate menopause/andropause symptoms. Effects are profound, dramatic and positive when done properly. Diet and lifestyle modification, such as implementing exercise 4 to 5 times a week, eating more plant-based, whole organic foods and avoiding processed foods, sugars and simple carbs. I will dive into these topics in the following chapters.

In my practice, the most common reasons women come to in to see me are: "I'm losing my hair!," "I'm losing my mind!," "I feel like I'm going crazy!," "I have no sex drive!" and "I'd rather sleep than worry about sex!" Women feel emotional, exhausted, "fat and puffy," and "sick of the nightmare hot flashes!" The most common reason I see men in my office, "I have no sex drive!," "My sex drive and erections just aren't the same, Doc!," "I'm exhausted and can't sleep!," and "I'm not the same person I used to be—I'm tired, having a hard time focusing, feel numb, and I hate my gut!"

Restoring hormones with BHRT doesn't alter your personality. It just makes you who you were on hormones. It is a refresher on how you felt before aging. You go back to who you, your spouse, kids, coworkers and friends remember you being. I advise my patients, as many are heavily distressed when they first start seeing me, not to make any life-altering decisions, such as marriage, divorce, quitting work or school, etc., until their hormones are balanced. When hormones are low or unbalanced, people tend to make "emotional" decisions and react emotionally, instead of logically. When a patient's hormones are restored and balanced, people tend to make "logical" decisions and react logically, not emotionally. God put our brain above our heart. It is important to use logic, followed by emotion. We are mammals and what makes mammals superior survivors and creatures is that we have a higher intellectual capacity. We need to use it as much as possible.

I especially tell people who have relationship conflicts, especially with their spouse or partner, not to focus on them. Focus on yourself, heal yourself, change yourself to become happy. Stop blaming others and look in the mirror to change your habits and lifestyle. Complaining about others is a distraction and an excuse not to fix oneself. Patients feel dramatically better after BHRT and are more sensitive, less blaming, more accountable and put forth much more effort toward their relationships after "feeling" more themselves and liking who they are again. They sleep better, exercise regularly, eat better, have improved sex drive and are more vibrant and happier. They most often inspire their spouse or partner to want to be better. It is most frequent in my practice that partners enthusiastically come in soon after for their own BHRT evaluation. They are motivated and hopeful after their spouse/partner transforms and grows younger!

It is important to remember that, when most couples get together, they usually have more hormones in place; by the time they evolve together, they both have probably depleted or greatly reduced their hormone stores. Both may feel exhausted, obese, have poor sleep and sex drives, and feel down, overwhelmed and sensitive. If there is a baseline LOVE, they need to restore their hormones—not find new lovers! That won't fix anything; it only makes things worse! They will just put a Band-Aid on things, not genuinely fix the real issues, just as a drug sustains a chronic disease, not cures it. By not restoring hormones, you will exhaust one relationship after another. Fix yourself and be accountable for how you feel and what you do.

ARE BIO-IDENTICAL HORMONES SAFE?

Yes, bio-identical hormones are safe because they are plant-based transdermal creams that are structurally identical to human hormones; the body recognizes them, binds to them, metabolizes them, and excretes them, activating the same functions as before andropause and menopause set in. Bio-identical hormones are plant-based, from soybeans or wild yams, are custom-compounded, with custom dosing and easy monitoring.

Bio-identical hormones have a half-life between 8 to 12 hours for estrogens, and about 24 hours for progesterone. Testosterone is also about 24 hours half-life. When you apply the hormones, they work; when you don't, your levels drop back down to your baseline levels. BHRT restores hormone balance, improves cellular communication and repair, improves the innate immune system and optimizes every organ function. They do not change your personality; restoring hormones makes you go back to who you were with hormones.

WHY ARE WOMEN AFRAID OF TAKING HORMONES?

In other decades, there was been a lot of controversy over hormone replacement therapy. It is important to clarify the confusion, so women feel comfortable and understand the differences between synthetic hormones and bio-identical hormones. Non-BHRT, or synthetic hormones, are not structurally identical to human hormones. They contain molecular differences that the body recognizes as foreign. Synthetic estrogen replacement, when given with progestin, a synthetic progesterone, has increased health risks.

In 2002, a large study, called the Women's Health Initiative (WHI), conducted a review of over 16,000 women to assess the effects of synthetic hormone replacement therapy (HRT). Women either were taking synthetic estrogen-only therapy or combined synthetic estrogen and progestin, a synthetic progesterone. The findings were astonishing.

The study revealed that postmenopausal women who used the combination of synthetic estrogen and progestin (Prempro) had a higher risk of breast cancer, heart attack, stroke and blood clots. It was a 26% increase in breast cancer risk, a 29% higher heart attack risk, and a 41% higher stroke risk than the control groups. This 8.5-year study was cut short to 5.2 years after risks exceeded the benefits of taking synthetic hormones, and many doctors immediately recommended that patents stop synthetic hormone replacement therapy. The group of patients on estrogen-only replacement had non-significant reduction in breast cancer and colon cancer but a significant reduction in hip fractures. It has been concluded from the WHI study that progestin (synthetic progesterone) appears to increase risk in breast cancer, not estrogen.

The North American Menopause Society put out a position statement on estrogen, saying, *"The benefits of hormonal therapy outweigh its risks in healthy peri-menopausal and early postmenopausal women with menopausal-related symptoms and a low baseline risk of stroke."*

DO BIO-IDENTICAL HORMONES CAUSE CANCER?

As discussed above, there is no evidence that bio-identical hormones cause cancer. They are natural, plant-based, identical in molecular structure to those of the human body and have generally not been linked to specific cases of cancer. Synthetic hormones have been linked to cancer. Thirteen studies document that synthetic progestin significantly increases estrogen-stimulated breast cell replication and growth. In contrast, seven studies show that bio-identical progesterone does not induce estrogen-stimulated breast cell proliferation. Numerous studies have reported an increased risk of breast cancer with the use of synthetic progestins whereas bio-identical progesterone has not been associated with increased risk of breast cancer. Research has revealed that bio-identical progesterone may decrease the risk of breast cancer.

A large study was published in the *Journal of Breast Cancer Research and Treatment* that concerned 80,000 postmenopausal women on HRT. The women were monitored for more than eight years. The results showed women who used estrogen in combination with synthetic progestins had a 69% increase of breast cancer, compared to women who hadn't used HRT. In contrast, the women who used bio-identical progesterone in combination with estrogen had no increased risk in breast cancer. Another study of 1,150 women who used bio-identical progesterone showed a reduced risk of breast cancer compared to their counterparts who didn't use the natural progesterone.

In 2004, another study from the *International Journal of Cancer* followed 31,451 postmenopausal women who were on hormone replacement therapy (HRT). They reported that women using estriol did not have an increased risk of breast cancer, compared to women who never used HRT. Another study from 1997 showed that breast cancer was reduced by 58% in women with the highest estriol levels compared to those with lowest estriol levels.

In 2009, Dr. Kent Holtorf and his medical team conducted a detailed review of over 200 clinical studies and published data on BHRT and conventional HRT. He concluded, *"Physiological data and clinical outcomes demonstrate that bio-identical hormones are associated with lower risks, including the risk of breast cancer and cardiovascular disease, and are more efficacious than their synthetic and animal-derived counterparts. Until evidence is found to the contrary, bio-identical hormones remain the preferred method of HRT."* He also went on to say, *"A thorough review of the medical literature clearly supports the claim that bio-identical hormones have some distinctly different, often opposite, physiological effects of their synthetic hormones. The medical literature demonstrates that BHRT is highly effective and carries a reduced, rather than an increased risk of breast cancer and cardiovascular disease."*

WHAT IS THE DIFFERENCE BETWEEN SYNTHETIC HORMONES (HRT) AND BIO-IDENTICAL HORMONES (BHRT)?

As discussed above, bio-identical hormones are identical to those naturally produced by our bodies. They bind to our body's receptors, like lock-and-key, causing fewer side effects. They are plant-based, usually wild yam, with a short half-life duration of action. Synthetic hormones are seen as foreign to our bodies. They are made from different species than us. Premarin (stands for pregnant mare's urine) is a synthetic estrogen from a horse's urine. Prempro is a synthetic estrogen from horse urine combined with a synthetic progesterone. Progestin and Provera are synthetic progesterones. These all differ in their molecular structure and don't bind in the lock-and-key-fit with our body's receptors, causing side effects throughout the body. Some of these side effects are detailed below. Based on physiological results and the clinical outcomes and side effects, current evidence supports that BHRT is safer than synthetic hormone replacement.

NATURAL TRANSDERMAL BHRT ESTROGENS AND PROGESTERONE VS. SYNTHETIC ORAL HRT ESTROGENS AND PROGESTINS

NATURAL ESTROGENS

The following describe the effects of natural estrogens:

- Lower inflammation and are antioxidants. They lower HsCRP and homocysteine levels. These are inflammation markers in the blood that are indicative of heart disease, stroke, dementia and blood clotting.
- Lower LDL, raise HDL, and are cardio-protective
- Vasodilate arteries and lower blood pressure
- Increase brain clarity, memory and brain function
- Improve mood and energy
- Decrease heart disease by 40–50%
- Have short half-life, leaving body quickly—about 12 hours

SYNTHETIC ESTROGENS

The following describe the effects of synthetic estrogrens:

- Increase inflammation, raise cardiac markers HsCRP and homocysteine
- Increase blood pressure
- Increase liver enzymes
- Associated with weight gain and food cravings
- Increase risk of blood clotting
- Increase depression and mood swings
- Increase triglycerides, increase bad fats

- Associated with brain fog
- Stay in body for months

NATURAL PROGESTERONE

The following describe the effects of natural progesterone:

- Decreases risk of blood clots
- Protects against heart disease, lowers bad cholesterol
- Lowers blood pressure
- Anti-inflammatory
- Natural diuretic
- Maintains healthy HDL levels
- Promotes natural calming effect
- Helps promote sleep
- Breast cancer protective
- Neuroprotective
- Endometrial protective
- Improves libido
- Pregnancy hormone
- Balances estrogen
- Forms new bone, prevents osteoporosis
- Improves mood and anxiety
- Improves sleep
- Short half-life, about 24 hours.
- Improves metabolism

SYNTHETIC PROGESTERONE (PROGESTINS)

The following describe the effects of synthetic progesterone, or progestins:

- Increased risk of blood clots
- Increased risk of breast cancer
- Increased weight gain
- Increased depression and anxiety
- Increased fluid retention
- Acne
- Rashes
- Headaches
- Increased LDL, lowered HDL
- Hair loss
- Decreased libido
- Increased blood pressure
- Thyroid imbalances
- Heart artery constriction

CHAPTER 5

Optimizing Hormones in Men

Every man desires to live long, but no man wishes to be old.

—Jonathan Swift

Joseph's Story

JOSEPH WAS 57 YEARS OLD WHEN HE FIRST CAME TO SEE ME. He had a medical history that included 18 years of type 2 diabetes, high blood pressure, high cholesterol, obesity, tiredness, poor sleep, poor sex drive and erection function with Viagra, and he was on cholesterol, diabetic and blood pressure medications for years. He had no early morning erections, no dreams during sleep, excessive daytime fatigue and hunger.

On initial blood work, he presented with low total and free testosterone, high cholesterol, high blood sugars and dehydration. I started him on therapeutic and customized levels of BHRT testosterone, DHEA, thyroid medications, vitamins and a weight training/cardio regimen. I asked him to give up sugars and dairy as well as eat organic plant-based foods and minimal organic meats.

He came back in 3.5 weeks, sleeping deeply, occasionally dreaming, having random early morning erections, much improved energy, a weight loss of eight pounds, and an improved sex drive. At ten weeks, we rechecked his blood work, and he had much improved cholesterol, blood pressure and blood sugars. We reduced Joe's blood pressure and cholesterol medications by half and reduced his diabetic medications. By now, he had lost 15 pounds, was working out an hour five times a week and had given up dairy, gluten and simple sugar foods. He was now sleeping solid, having frequent early morning erections, improved erection quality, and having sex three times a week without Viagra. He was ecstatic, feeling stronger, more focused and had great energy and sex drive. He came back at six months, off blood pressure and cholesterol medications. Joe was taking only vitamins, working out consistently, and controlling his diabetes by diet only. No more medications, on medical grade vitamins, exercising, eating whole foods, on BHRT and feeling 20 years younger!

ERECTILE DYSFUNCTION

The most important intervention I do in my practice is prevent and evaluate for cardiac problems. When treating men with BHRT, remember, we reduce cardiac disease up to 40% by increasing blood supply to the heart, increasing cardiac output, lowering bad cholesterol and lowering blood pressure and blood sugars. The heart is a muscle, so is the penis. Both are innervated by nerves and blood vessels. The heart is the most important muscle although some men may beg to differ and propose that distinction is held by the penis.

When erection quality is poor, that means heart health is poor. That is a red flag. I believe in, first and foremost, fix the heart. When there is poor erection quality, this often means heart disease—either high cholesterol, high blood sugar or high blood pressure. When you "fix" the heart, you fix the penis. Prescribing the "blue pill" (Viagra or another), without evaluating heart health, is just a temporary Band-Aid effect covering up a serious underlying cardiac issue. When a man is low on testosterone, he has high blood sugar and cholesterol, which creates thick blood, like maple syrup, resulting in a traffic jam in the arteries, causing high blood pressure and slow blood flow. Arteries supply oxygen to the heart, brain, penis and every organ along the way.

When you optimize the hormones testosterone and thyroid, you turn the traffic jam in the blood vessels into a free-flowing speedway. The lanes are wider, there's less blood sugars and cholesterol blocking the pathway, blood viscosity turns more water-like, fast and easy flowing, resulting in lower blood pressure and more oxygen and blood to the heart, brain and penis. Testosterone also sustains muscle strength. Improved cardiac health means improved erection quality. This is a safe, natural way to recover and achieve superior erection quality and sexual satisfaction. *Happy Heart=Happy Penis.*

DOES TESTOSTERONE CAUSE PROSTATE CANCER RISK?

The majority of evidence indicates that testosterone does not cause prostate cancer. Prostate cancer does not occur in young 20-year-old men with high testosterone levels. Testosterone protects prostate size and function. As men age and have lower testosterone levels, the prostate grows. Low testosterone and high estrogen are associated with prostate cancer. Many studies have substantiated that TRT (testosterone replacement treatment) is not associated with an increase in prostate cancer. Studies show that older men with the highest risk of prostate cancer have the lowest serum testosterone levels. Low free testosterone actually correlated with positive prostate biopsy in one study. They also found in the same study decreasing testosterone was a risk factor for prostate cancer and high testosterone did not correlate with prostate specific antigen, or PSA.

Dr. Adam Morgenthaler, who has extensively studied and published on this relationship, broke the "T causes prostate cancer" myth. He concluded, *"There is not now—nor has there ever been—a scientific basis for the belief that testosterone causes prostate cancer to grow."* However, men with active prostate cancer should not take TRT.

WHAT REDUCES BPH (BENIGN PROSTATE HYPERTROPHY) AND PROSTATE CANCER?

- Ideal body weight
- Saw Palmetto
- Frequent sex
- Diet high in vegetables and plant-based foods
- Avoidance of smoking and excessive alcohol
- Green tea
- Fiber: 25–35 grams a day
- Zinc citrate
- Curcumin
- Vitamin C
- DIM (diindolylmethane)

Zinc

Zinc is critical for preserving prostate health in men. Zinc helps inhibit testosterone conversion to estrogen. The prostate needs 10 times more zinc than any other organ in the body. It tends to be poorly absorbed in the body; men after 65 years old only absorb half the zinc they used to absorb at 30 years. Alcohol reduces zinc levels in the body. Zinc deficiency is associated with hair loss, eczema, poor immune system, frequent viral infections, poor wound healing and impotency.

What Are the Greatest Risk Factors for Prostate Cancer?

- 55 years or older
- Father with prostate cancer or mother with breast cancer
- High estrogen levels
- Obesity
- Zinc deficiency

- Alcohol abuse
- High DHT (dihydrotestosterone, a byproduct of testosterone)

MEN AND ESTROGEN

Estrogen is not just a female hormone. Men have a small fraction of estrogen that helps maintain brain health and bone density. However, too much estrogen in men can displace testosterone of its receptor sites and cause negative effects. Estrogen levels must be monitored in men. The ratio of testosterone to estrogen is more significant than absolute estrogen levels. The average 60-year-old man has higher blood estrogen levels than a 60-year-old female. With andropause, men's testes stop producing testosterone, and estrogen levels rise due to fat cells releasing more estrogen. An enzyme called aromatase, found mostly in fat cells, can convert testosterone into estrogen. Estrogen is the first derivative of testosterone. As we grow older and gain more fat, aromatase activity increases, and estrogen levels rise. Studies have shown higher levels of estrogen in men directly correlate to more thickening in the carotid artery lining, which increases risk of strokes and heart disease. High estrogen in men can also cause gynecomastia (male breast tissue), low sex drive, increased fat tissue, increased risk of diabetes and BPH (benign prostate hypertrophy) and is linked to prostate cancer.

Estrogen in men rises with aging, obesity, a high-fat diet, excessive alcohol use, marijuana use, GMOs and environmental toxins, and zinc deficiency. Certain medications, using high levels of injectable testosterone, and having high levels of cortisol from chronic stressors all cause estrogen levels to rise. Some common medications that are known to increase estrogen levels in men are cholesterol-lowering drugs, some blood pressure meds, antacids, over-the-counter anti-inflammatory meds, anti-depressants, antibiotics, and antifungal meds. Alcohol has been shown to reduce zinc levels and significantly inhibit estrogen clearance from the body.

BHRT for men, weight loss, avoiding alcohol, resistance training 2 to 3 times a week, eating a diet full of cruciferous vegetables and taking supplements like zinc, vitamin C, chrysin, and DIM will stimulate the removal of excess estrogen. Zinc helps inhibit testosterone conversion to estrogen. Monitoring estrogen, along with testosterone levels, helps prevent disease and extends a man's quality of life.

WHAT IS SARCOPENIA?

Sarcopenia, loss of skeletal muscle mass, causes frailty. Frailty is a consequence of aging and is a major health concern. Fragility is actually a medical condition. It consists of unwanted weight loss, weakness, slow walking speed, self-reported exhaustion and less physical activity. Fragility also poses a risk for osteoporosis and bone fractures. BHRT for men and women helps prevent sarcopenia. BHRT along with weight-strengthening exercising improves muscle mass and strength.

CHAPTER 6

Optimizing Hormones in Women

Nature gives you the face you have at twenty;
it's up to you to merit the face you have at fifty.

—Coco Chanel

Jennifer's Story

JENNIFER WAS A 42-YEAR OLD WOMAN. SHE CAME TO ME FEELING tired even though she worked out, she was sensitive and hyper-emotional, and her hair was dry, shedding and not growing. She was losing her sex drive and orgasms; she was having a hard time feeling sexy or even thinking about sex. She had a history of an endometrial ablation, a strong family history of breast cancer, heart disease and diabetes, and felt like she was much older than she was. She felt "puffy." She worked out regularly and was frustrated she was not losing weight. She had low self-esteem—and no matter what she bought, it didn't make her feel pretty or confident enough. She was missing her confidence, feeling tired and vulnerable.

Jennifer would say, *"The doctors keep telling me I'm normal, the labs are all normal, but I just don't feel good! I'm working out, eating right and not losing weight! I feel puffy, and my hair is thinning, dry and won't grow."*

Upon doing her blood work, Jennifer's labs came back positive for Hashimoto thyroiditis, which is very common in perimenopausal women. I balanced Jennifer's thyroid levels, modified her nutrition and restored her "gut" health by eliminating gluten and dairy, and drastically cutting down on wine, sugar and all simple carbs. We reviewed different ways of stress management and improved work-out methods by incorporating resistance training. Within weeks, Jennifer felt improvement in her sleep, sex drive, vaginal lubrication, yeast infections, and UTIs with Bio-identical Hormones. Within months, Jennifer felt much more confident, sexy, strong, beautiful, and loved her age and body. She had her sex drive and orgasms back. Jennifer feels younger than when she first came to me; she's been with me 10 years now and looks and feels better than ever! She, like many other patients, reports at her follow-up visits, *"I feel great, Doc!"*

WOMEN WITH SURGICAL-INDUCED MENOPAUSE, ENDOMETRIAL ABLATIONS AND HYSTERECTOMIES

Sandra's Story

Sandra was 48 years old and suffering from constant hot flashes during the day and night sweats throughout the night. Six months previously, she had a total hysterectomy. Although she is relieved she has no more irregular, heavy, clot-filled periods, she now suffers from 15 pounds of weight gain, frequent headaches, daily hot flashes, night sweats, poor sleep, poor sex drive, fatigue, dry vaginal skin, muscle aches and pains, and brain fog. She complains about feeling more depressed, anxious and is very emotional. Upon telling her regular doctor, Sandra was offered an antidepressant and anti-anxiety medications. She didn't feel comfortable taking either, so she didn't.

On her first visit with me, after a complete evaluation and review of labs, Sandra was started on a customized BHRT, supplements and a modified nutrition plan avoiding dairy, sugar and simple carbs. After one week, I asked her to start walking 40 minutes, five times a week. Sandra came back in one month later to report, *"I feel so much better, Doc! No more hot flashes!"* She had barely any hot flashes, no more night sweats, improved sleep, was dreaming once in a while, woke up with more energy, had improved vaginal lubrication, no more headaches, fewer muscle aches, and was feeling less depressed and anxious. After two months, Sandra was thrilled to report her brain fog had lifted, her sex drive was better, and she was walking regularly and losing weight. Sandra's skin was visibly more radiant—and so was she.

After a total hysterectomy (meaning the removal of the uterus and ovaries), a woman goes into full-blown menopause and feels the symptoms immediately. With partial hysterectomies (meaning the ovaries are spared), a woman feels less symptomatic. In my practice, I have noticed that women with histories of uterine ablations and partial hysterectomies are more prone to menopausal symptoms earlier if they don't have healthy diets, exercise regularly or sleep properly. They tend to experience weight gain, headaches, fatigue, poor sleep and poor sex drive sooner. Most women with ablations and hysterectomies are relieved to have no more painful, heavy periods. However, they have new symptoms that they hadn't expected. Research shows that about 60–70% of women, even with their ovaries left, feel a decrease in hormones within 3 to 4 years of their operation. During their surgery, the uterine artery is cut and tied off, so the ovaries get less blood perfusion and they produce less hormones.

According to the CDC, about 600,000 hysterectomies are performed in the U.S. every year. About one-third of American women have had hysterectomies. This means all these women will suffer higher risks of menopausal symptoms, especially with increased cardiac risk factors, not to mention hot flashes, obesity, insomnia, poor sex drive and brain fog. BHRT provides these women with natural, healing hormones to relieve their suffering and restore their health and vitality.

WHAT IS ESTROGEN DOMINANCE?

Dr. John R. Lee coined the term "estrogen dominance," explaining that it is a state of a woman with little, normal or too high estrogen but little or no progesterone to balance estrogen's effects. This could happen at any age. Examples of estrogen dominance include polycystic ovarian syndrome (PCOS) and peri/postmenopausal women. So, even in a low estrogen state, like menopause, women can be estrogen dominant. Dr. Lee explained that progesterone is important, and without a healthy, balanced level of progesterone, estrogen dominates. Estrogen and progesterone work together in the body. A healthy estrogen-to-progesterone ratio is critical for balance and well-being.

Some common reasons for estrogen imbalance are environmental toxins, poor diet and nutrition, stress that over-stimulates the adrenal glands to release high cortisol, poor gut health and obesity. Obesity creates imbalance and danger for excessive endogenous estrogen production. Fat cells release E1. The more obese the person, the more endogenous fat cell release of estrogen, creating a large imbalance of estrogen to progesterone, leading to estrogen dominance. Chronic stress lowers progesterone production and increases cortisol production, leading to estrogen dominance. Environmental toxins can be in our foods, makeup, water, and plastic products like water bottles, cooking tools, cleaning agents and fragrances. These toxins are called xenoestrogens; they release estrogen mimickers of E1 into the body creating an unhealthy estrogen dominance. They are "estrogen-like" chemicals and toxins associated with cancers and disease because they disrupt proper estrogen balance by binding to the body's estrogen receptors and triggering abnormal effects. The progesterone-to-estrogen ratio diminishes.

There is a higher risk of breast cancer, uterine cancer, heavy periods with abnormal bleeding, and infertility issues in women with a high estrogen-to-progesterone ratio. Remember, hormones are team players; they have to work in harmony to keep the body optimally healthy. It is a complex interaction. The wrong hormone balance accelerates aging and disease. The right progesterone-to-estrogen ratio helps manage and slow down aging and disease process.

Treatments discussed in detail in this book include managing stress better, switching to clean makeup, switching to grass-fed, pasture-raised organic produce, meat and eggs, and eating mostly a high-fiber, plant-based diet. Also included is improving sleep quality and implementing exercise four times a week to lose weight and burn fat. Thyroid hormones have to be evaluated to assure weight loss and optimal function. Taking supplements (that will be discussed in later chapters) can help, such as DIM, B complex, system enzymes, probiotics, fiber, vitamin D3, and resveratrol.

WOMEN AND TESTOSTERONE

Testosterone is produced in the ovaries and adrenal glands in women. Testosterone helps to maintain muscle tone, memory, cognition and confidence, and it decreases body fat and helps maintain a healthy sex drive for both men and women. Low levels of testosterone in women are associated with poor sex drive, poor self-esteem, weight gain, reduced bone mass, brain fog, poor muscle tone, and thinning skin and hair. High testosterone levels, which usually occur with menopause, can also occur during puberty and midlife, with PCOS (polycystic ovarian syndrome). High testosterone levels can cause acne, aggression, hirsutism (excessive facial and body hair, male hair distribution), diabetes, and an increased risk of heart disease.

In order to have testosterone's positive effects on the heart and brain, its impact on lowering heart disease and its ability to increase memory and confidence, it's important to optimize BHRT estrogen in women. Research shows postmenopausal women who get BHRT testosterone have an increase in sex drive, response, sexual satisfaction, sexual fantasies, sexual frequency and sexual arousal. Testosterone improves a woman's clitoral and nipple sensitivity and improves orgasm quality. This is a huge relief to many women who lose their sex drive during perimenopause and menopause. BHRT testosterone also increases muscle tone and skin tone, decreases body fat and maintains bone strength.

CHAPTER 7

Youthful Skin Secrets

Youth is happy because it has the capacity to see beauty.
Anyone who keeps the ability to see beauty never grows old.

—Franz Kafka

THE SKIN IS THE LARGEST ORGAN OF OUR BODY. OUR SKIN IS A canvas of the inflammation we carry in our body. It is a reflection of how we eat, hydrate, sleep, exercise, think, balance our hormones, and cope with stress. The key to having great skin is having great gut health. Doing the things above fix and maintain optimal gut health.

Our skin indicates what's happening inside our gut and body. People spend insane amounts of money on superficial fixes and plastic surgery. I advise fixing the skin from the inside out. Then fine-tune what you desire, and the results will be much more satisfying. The aging population is increasing, so it is no surprise that the vast amount of anti-aging products and procedures are targeted at women. I believe in maximizing our confidence and youth while re-energizing our skin. However, it starts with optimizing our hormones and lifestyle, which will allow the facial products we use to be more effective, and plastic surgery to be more limited and satisfying (if you so choose).

HOW TO RE-ENERGIZE AND REJUVENATE YOUR SKIN

Aging is a fact of life. Looking your age is not.

—Dr. Howard Murad

1. BHRT—Restoring and balancing hormones is a powerful step in reversing aging skin. BHRT for both men and women improves skin quality by slowing down collagen loss, increasing collagen production, increasing skin turnover and improving the skin's ability to retain water and moisture.

After 30 years old, collagen production drops 1% every year. Skin is also made up of ceramides, a fat layer on the top layer of the skin that forms a barrier to protect the skin and retain skin moisture. They naturally decrease with age. By age 30, we lose about 40%, and by age 40, we lose up to a staggering 60%! Estrogen affects skin moisture, wrinkle formation, and skin thickness. Estrogen increases glycosaminoglycans (GAGs), such as hyaluronic acid, a natural "skin filler." Hyaluronic acids maintain fluid balance and structural integrity of the skin. Estrogen can also increase ceramide and collagen production of the outer skin layer to keep skin plump, hydrated and wrinkle-free.

After starting my patents on customized BHRT, there is a dramatic improvement in skin quality in both sexes. Before BHRT, skin is generally, itchy, sensitive, thin, dry and pale, with more fine wrinkles. Restoring it with BHRT hormones shows in the face almost immediately with thicker, tighter, better hydrated skin with improved tone and color. Skin also looks brighter, not sallow or dull. The hormones are critical for preventing further wrinkles and sagging. Just a little hormone fine-tuning makes a big difference.

Many women get skin pigmentation, called melasma, a hormone-related skin discoloration. Melasma is usually on the face when exposed to sun or on the cheeks, nose or forehead. This condition is usually from hormone fluctuations, like too much estrogen during pregnancy, or is due to some oral contraceptive use, loss of estrogen or menopause. In my experience, replacing estrogen in

BHRT, melasma can be minimized, greatly reduced and prevented. Women still need to avoid excessive direct sun exposure and wear sunscreen.

2. NUTRITION—Our skin reflects how we eat. Eating abundant organic vegetables, fruits, fish, eggs, nuts, olives, avocados, seeds, sprouted grains and moderate amounts of organic, grass-fed meats produce great skin. Soda, alcohol and excessive coffee, refined carbs, simple sugars, processed foods, fast food, animal meats filled with preservatives, fats like dairy and cheese, and GMO-grown foods are not good for the skin. Sugar is an age accelerator; it ages our skin and causes wrinkles. Sugar should be from fruits and consumed in all-natural forms. Refined sugar should be avoided as much as possible. Sugar creates inflammation, insulin resistance and diabetes, and causes thinning of skin collagen, deep wrinkling and sagging skin. High sugar levels cross-link with collagen, called glycation, and decrease its elasticity and strength, forming deep facial grooves.

3. PROPER HYDRATION—A well-hydrated intact skin barrier is critical to make skin look naturally plump and youthful. Drink half your body weight in ounces daily of "active" alkaline water.

4. EXERCISE—Working out is also essential for improved skin quality. Sweating during exercising detoxes, cleanses the pores and increases circulation to the skin. Working out—especially cardio and resistance training—revs up your own hormone production; it releases HGH, the ultimate anti-aging hormone, as discussed earlier, that pumps up collagen production, producing a natural glow. HGH, estrogen and testosterone all restore collagen fibers that naturally tone, tighten and lift the skin.

5. GUT HEALTH—Years of eating too much sugar and refined carbs, as we've learned, destroys our good bacteria and ruins our gut health. Eating a diet full of vegetables and whole organic foods fixes our gut health. We wear our gut health on our skin. Good gut flora=good skin flora. So, take a probiotic every day, along with eating organic whole foods.

6. SUPPLEMENTATION—A probiotic and omega-3 fish oils are best for skin. I also recommend vitamin C with bioflavonoids called ester C to boost collagen production, brighten skin, and even out skin tone. In the chapter to come on supplementation, I review in detail antioxidants and anti-inflammatory vitamins. They are amazing powerhouses to rejuvenate and transform the body and skin to vibrant health and youth!

7. BEAUTY SLEEP—Sleep 7 to 8 hours a night. Researchers from a Scotland study reported sleep deprivation causes skin to age faster. *"This research shows, for the first time, that poor sleep quality can accelerate signs of skin aging and weaken the skin's ability to repair itself at night,"* Dr. Daniel Yarosh reported after the study made a positive connection between sleep and skin aging. During deep sleep, growth hormone is released, which repairs damaged cells and preserves moisture, glow and collagen. Poor sleep and sleep deprivation release the stress hormone cortisol, which leads to inflammation, poor skin quality and a dehydrated, dry, flaky, dull complexion and breakouts. Increased cortisol over time increases inflammatory skin conditions such as acne and psoriasis. Sleep is so important to have youthful, glowing and bright skin.

8. SKIN PRODUCTS—I recommend using only natural products for your face and neck. That means no parabens, sulfates, mineral oil, synthetic fragrances or colors, silicones or glycols—try to get all your products without these chemicals. I recommend avoiding washing with hot water, and gentle exfoliating no more than twice a week, as overuse strips away the microbiomes and all the protective oils in the skin. I recommend applying a plant-based natural retinol daily at night, which increases collagen production and reduces pigmentation. Use a natural eye cream day and night, along with an oil cleanser, toner and moisturizer. Using invigorating essential oils, such as rosehip oil or Marula oil, hydrates, improves elasticity and reinforces the outer lipid barrier of the skin. Finally, use a natural sunscreen on your neck and face daily.

CHAPTER 8

Benefits of Hormonal Balance

Aging is an extraordinary process where you become
the person you always should have been.
—David Bowie

BALANCING OUR HORMONES ALLOW US TO AGE MORE SLOWLY, sleep better, be happier, feel confident, gain muscle, burn fat, have a stronger sex drive and have more satisfying sex. Men and women both feel younger, more energized and emotionally balanced. They have more energy to work out and eat healthier. Balancing our hormones is a critical step to attaining optimal overall health.

Our life should be rich in hormones, not just the first third of our life, for our entire lifespan! Bio-identical hormone restoration lets us experience the full joy of life by recharging our immune system and preserving our skin, brain, heart and gut health. They safely reprogram us back into a youthful state, by preserving a positive mental attitude, allowing us to be motivated to work out, think harder, feel deeper, smile and laugh harder, sleep deeper, restore your sex drive and tap into powerful orgasms, cope with stress better and lose weight easier.

Bio-identical hormones protect us from aging faster than we have to due to environment, poor lifestyle choices and accelerated depletion of hormones from stress. In the following chapters, I will discuss how hormone balancing along with a healthy lifestyle, vital nutrition and high-grade vitamins, can all play a huge role in our life extension, gene modification and stem cell preservation. Life is sacred—we have to be proactive to preserve it.

Bio-identical hormones safely allow us to transform from a state of decaying, aging and degenerating to powerful state of protective regenerating youth, with vigor and ease!

PART II

NUTRITION

CHAPTER 9

Optimizing Nutrition Is the Key to a Healthier You

Let food be thy medicine and medicine be thy food.

—Hippocrates

THERE ARE SO MANY FAD DIETS BOMBARDING OUR SOCIETY and social media. What is the best diet plan? I recommend that just as we customize BHRT for people, we should customize a food plan as well. A food plan is *a daily plan*, a lifestyle for life. Generally, low sugar intake, high plant-based proteins and foods, minimum animal fat proteins, and a high good fat diet. Two of the healthiest diets in the world, time-tested and validated by hundreds of studies, which I strongly support and educate my patients about, are the traditional Mediterranean and Okinawan diets. Both diets are nutrient-rich, loaded with seasonal vegetables, fruit, nuts, legumes, seafood, limited animal proteins, adequate water intake and limited alcohol. I will discuss in this chapter how we can use Mother Nature's foods to heal ourselves from illness and diseases caused mostly by environmental toxins and overconsumption of poor-quality foods.

To begin with, it is important to rule out allergies or sensitivities to dairy and gluten. Gluten means "glue" in Latin and is the protein usually found in wheat, rye, oats, barley and spelt. It's a food additive that binds together breads, cakes, doughnuts, pizza dough, crackers, and just about anything made with flour, to make it chewy, soft and stretchy. Gluten is added into processed foods, sauces, condiments, drinks and even personal care products, like makeup, hair conditioners, lotions, and so much more. A blood test is an easy way to detect these in your system. If you have severe abdominal pain, gas, bloating, diarrhea or constipation, and headaches when eating gluten, additional blood and genetic testing to evaluate for celiac disease may be needed. Celiac disease is a hereditary autoimmune disorder. The treatment is to eat a strict gluten-free diet.

Many people with thyroid conditions tend to be gluten- and dairy-sensitive and do much better when they avoid gluten and dairy foods, since both are pro-inflammatory foods. Most gluten foods are rich in simple sugars and GMO-made. Dr. Perlmutter, renowned neurologist and author of *The Grain Brain*, brilliantly details how gluten in simple carbohydrates inflames not just the gut, but the entire brain and body. This is an excellent book I recommend to many of my patients to help them learn how bad refined sugars, flours and gluten are for our bodies.

I recommend to most patients with autoimmune disorders that they avoid pro-inflammatory foods: gluten, processed carbohydrates, simple sugars and dairy. Eating whole organic vegetables, fruits, free-range meats and eggs, nuts, seeds and grains provides a richer anti-inflammatory diet.

Unfortunately, the standard American diet is low in whole-plant foods, high in animal fat, sugar and salt, and low in fiber.

OBESITY=HIGH INFLAMMATION=CHRONIC DISEASE=CANCER!!!

Obesity is the number one health problem in the United States. It is also a global problem. In 1980, there were 250 million obese people worldwide. In 2008, the rate rose to 904 million people! The prevalence of obesity has been rising over the last 50 years. Presently, greater than two-thirds of adults and one-third of kids and teens are overweight or obese. People are eating calorie-rich and nutrient-poor foods, which explains why an astounding 70% of the U.S. adult population is overweight or obese. Obesity is linked with heart disease, stroke, type 2 diabetes, infertility, joint and back pain, and cancer. Type 2 diabetes, due to poor eating, lack of exercise and obesity, has become a national epidemic. Almost 90% of type 2 diabetics are overweight or obese at the time of diagnosis.

In a 2016 study published in *The New England Journal of Medicine* reviewing 1,000 other studies, researchers concluded that there is *"sufficient evidence to link weight gain, overweight and obesity with 13 cancers."* They included pancreas, kidney, thyroid, multiple myeloma, meningioma, stomach, esophagus, colon and rectal, liver, gallbladder, uterus, ovarian, and breast cancers. Also, revealed in the Nurses' Health Study, *"an 18-year follow-up of almost 93,000 women, a dose-response association of weight gain and obesity with several cancers."* This means that there is a direct relationship between increased weight gain and obesity with an increased cancer risk. The researchers also noted childhood obesity most often leads to adult obesity.

Obesity is a risk factor for cancer because obesity increases inflammation, raises insulin levels and raises the abnormal sex hormone E1 that is released from fat cells into the blood. These abnormal estrogens cause cancer cells to grow unchecked.

Research has also shown that obesity causes alteration of the gut permeability, leading to leaky gut syndrome, which lowers the potential of the innate immune system, leading to a cascade of inflammation, disease and cancer formation.

Successful lifestyle modification reduces obesity, inflammation and disease progression. Obesity is preventable and reversible. Checking and balancing your entire hormone profile, especially thyroid function, walking one hour daily, eating plant-based proteins and foods, and avoiding dairy, animal fats and foods, soda, sugar, alcohol, simple carbohydrates and processed foods are imperative. Also, taking probiotics, vitamin D3, curcumin, resveratrol and other supplements—as elaborated on in later chapters—and properly hydrating with water (half your body weight in ounces daily) are equally important.

CHAPTER 10

Gut Health Is Everything!

All disease begins in the gut.

—Hippocrates

BACTERIA HAVE BEEN THE TARGETS OF MEDICINE FOR centuries. Louis Pasteur, a famous French chemist from the 1850s, developed pasteurization, which is the killing of bacteria with heat. He also discovered principles of vaccination to stop bacterial contamination. Soon after, in the 1940s, Alexander Fleming discovered the antibiotic—penicillin—to kill bacteria. Since then, when used properly, these antibiotics have saved lives daily. They either kill bacteria or prevent them from reproducing. Unfortunately, overuse and easy access of antibiotics have led to the destruction of our healthy gut flora.

The word itself, "anti" means "against" and "bios" means "life" so "antibiotic" means "against life." An antibiotic kills bacteria when we take it, without distinguishing between the good and bad bacteria. The good bacteria, gut flora, or intestinal bacteria is destroyed along with the invading bacterium. We have good bacteria, from our oral opening all the way down to our rectum. Frequent side effects like heartburn, diarrhea and upset stomach occur when the good bacteria is killed. This is why a probiotic supplement is important when it is necessary to take antibiotics. A probiotic will sustain the balance of good bacteria to bad bacteria. Other reasons a healthy microbiome gets imbalanced can be poor diet, toxins and an unhealthy lifestyle.

"Pro" means "for," and "bios" means "life," so "probiotic" means "for life." Probiotics promote and restore the growth of our internal good bacteria. One of the probiotics, lactobacillus, inhibits the growth of H. pylori, a microbe responsible for 90% of stomach ulcers, and eventually stomach cancer if left untreated. Probiotics prevent C. difficile, a bacteria triggered by antibiotic use, that could cause a potentially severe, life-threatening diarrhea.

Our skin and the digestive tract are covered with trillions of healthy bacteria and yeast, which is also called microbiome. We have the greatest amount of this healthy bacteria in our digestive tract, especially the small intestine. A healthy adult gut should have between 2 to 3 pounds of good bacteria, about 100 trillion organisms. We are one big symbiotic organism.

Within the small intestine is located Peyer's Patches, which is responsible for 70–80% of the immune system! That means our immune system depends on our internal good bacteria outweighing bad bacteria. A healthy gut is critical to have a healthy immune system.

The intestinal wall in the gut has more nerve endings than the spinal cord. This is called the enteric nervous system. Neuroscientific research shows the digestive tract is actually responsible for producing 90% of the body's serotonin! Serotonin is the "happy endorphin" responsible for feeling happy, fighting depression, controlling appetite and inducing deep sleep. GABA (gamma-Aminobutyric acid) is also released by a healthy gut microbiome. GABA naturally promotes calm and prevents anxiety in our body. Melatonin, a natural sleep inducer and a potent antioxidant, is also released by healthy gut flora. This is called the "gut-brain axis." The gut is, in a sense, our "second brain." This is profound, and it is absolutely critical to appreciate this connection between gut and brain. We need to preserve, restore and protect our healthy gut bacteria on a daily basis to preserve our immune system and mental health.

A diet low in sugar and high in vegetables, active cultured foods, fiber and water helps grow probiotics naturally. Sugar, food toxins (such as GMOs), stress, foods high in animal fat proteins and dairy, soda, excessive alcohol, artificial sweeteners, and antibiotics kill the body's own good gut probiotics. NSAIDS (non-steroidal anti-inflammatory drugs) such as aspirin, Motrin, Aleve, acetamino-phen, Tylenol, birth control pills, prednisone, along with a myriad of prescription drugs, also damage a healthy gut. I have found in my practice that processed wheat products, or gluten (wheat, barley, rye and oats), and processed dairy and GMO corn and soy products also kill off good bacteria. Gluten is the "glue" food additive that sticks to the gut lining, interferes and prevents the breakdown and absorption of nutrients. This leaves a thick, gluey, pasty, poorly digested residue in the gut.

When bad bacteria exceed good bacteria, dysbiosis results. Dysbiosis is a damaged gut flora, also known as "leaky gut." The gut lining is a long tube with tight protective barriers and tight cell junctions like a zipper. A leaky gut has damaged cell junctions. It has holes in the lining, like a broken zipper, so there is poor absorption of food and nutrients, leading to nutritional deficiencies. With a damaged gut flora and low good bacteria, regular bowel movements are more difficult.

With a damaged and leaky gut, allergens and undigested food particles slip through the GI (gastrointestinal) tract, enter the bloodstream and cause inflammation in the body. Also, in a leaky gut, invasion of the gut by viruses, bacteria, yeast and toxins occurs. This also leads to chronic inflammation and food intolerances, and the body is unable to breakdown toxins to excrete into stool. Scientists have now found that these food intolerances cause the body to chronically inflame (also known as chronic inflammation) and start producing antibodies against itself. This starts an autoimmune process and, eventually, an autoimmune disease. Leaky gut syndrome has been linked to autoimmune diseases. However, by reestablishing the gut barrier function with probiotic supplementation, we may reverse or dramatically improve the autoimmune process and disease.

Scientists have strong evidence connecting dysbiosis to obesity, heart disease, type 2 diabetes, major depression, anxiety, schizophrenia, Alzheimer's, Parkinson's, autism, ADD, ADHD, irritable bowel syndrome and colorectal cancer. Tooth decay, gum disease and seasonal allergies are also connected to an imbalanced gut health.

New research at San Francisco State University has shown that cardiovascular exercise can boost gut health by increasing the good bacteria in the gut microbiome. The study tracked students who worked out on the treadmill and those who didn't. Subjects maintained food logs, and gut bacteria from their stool samples were analyzed. Those students with higher fitness levels had higher levels of firmicutes bacteris, a healthy gut bacterium that prevents leaky gut syndrome. Lead researcher Ryan Durk reported, *"We now know that exercise is crucial for increasing beneficial bacteria in the gut."*

Research strongly supports that a healthy gut protects us from cancers, allergies, diabetes, heart disease and psychiatric illnesses. Healthy gut flora is critical for brain health, heart health and immune system strength. Leaky gut=brain fog and a poor immune system.

For parents raising children with autism, depression, ADD, ADHD or schizophrenia, or adults who have these conditions, a great book to read that explains the gut/brain connection is Dr. Natasha Campbell-McBride's *Gut and Psychology Syndrome*. It is an excellent book that I recommend to my patients to help themselves or their affected children.

Most fascinating is Louis Pasteur's deathbed confession in 1895, *"I have been wrong. The germ is nothing. The terrain is everything."*

HOW DO YOU GET SUPERIOR GUT HEALTH?

1. Cut out processed foods, sugars, gluten and dairy by at least 80%, if not entirely, if you are more sensitive or allergic.

2. Take a medical-grade probiotic.

3. Balance your hormones. Balanced and restored estrogen, testosterone and thyroid hormones promote healthy gut bacteria (while high cortisol destroys healthy gut bacteria and creates inflammation and dysbiosis).

4. Eat foods rich in glutamine and quercetin. Glutamine is an essential amino acid that promotes gut healing. Examples of glutamine-rich foods are cabbage, broccoli, Brussels sprouts, and raw goat milk. Try not to overcook these foods; just flash steam the food or, even more potent, is to eat it raw. Quercetin is a powerful bioflavonoid, meaning it's a strong antioxidant that lowers inflammation, thereby repairing dysbiosis. It is found in onions, apples, red wine and green tea. Quercetin also chelates heavy metals, meaning it breaks them down and detoxes them from your body.

5. Eat organic, whole foods with high fiber: vegetables, fruits and meat.

6. Eat fermented foods, such as sauerkraut, kimchi, organic yogurt or kefir. They have high glutamine content too.

7. Take a curcumin supplement or cook with the spice turmeric. Turmeric is the yellow Indian spice that is rich in curcumin and used by cooks for centuries. It is a powerful antioxidant that helps lower inflammation throughout the entire body, especially helpful with restoring good bacteria in the gut.

8. Regular exercise, which will be detailed in chapters to come, has been proven to increase good gut bacterial growth and improve gut microbiome.

9. Take vitamin D3 to boost your innate immune system to ward off infections and to prevent having to take antibiotics.

10. Eat more prebiotic foods, explained further below.

Function of Probiotics

Following are the functions of probiotics (friendly bacteria):

- Maintains the integrity of the gut lining
- Balances the gut pH
- Helps in digestion and absorption of essential nutrients
- Makes IgA—an immunoglobulin from mother's breast milk that fights viruses
- Regulates the immune system

- Produces essential vitamins like K and biotin
- Absorbs and excretes carcinogenic byproducts into the stool
- Suppresses the hyperplastic process in the gut, a process of cancer formation
- Neutralizes toxins and chemicals, and chelates heavy metals into the stool
- Keeps bowel movements regular
- Regulates the neurological system
- Acts as a natural internal antibiotic, antiviral and antifungal
- Food sources: pickles, olives, sauerkraut, kimchi, organic tempeh, miso soup, sourdough bread, yogurt, dark chocolate, kombucha

Function of Prebiotics

Following are the functions of prebiotics:

- Acts as food for probiotics
- Supports and nourishes probiotic growth
- Ensures the growth and increases the number of probiotic bacteria
- Derived from carbohydrates rich in fibers
- Food sources: berries, bananas, cherries, kiwi, artichokes, asparagus, garlic, leeks, onions, leafy rich greens, lentils, chickpeas, black and white beans, flaxseed, quinoa, oatmeal, raw walnuts, chia seeds, flaxseeds and ocean-based plants like chlorella, spirulina and blue-green algae

Our gut health is a huge player in our overall heath. A healthy gut bolsters our immune system, prevents disease and maximizes nutrient absorption.

CHAPTER 11

Organic Foods vs. Conventional GMO Foods

Children today are sicker than they were a generation ago.
From childhood cancers to autism, birth defects and asthma,
a wide range of childhood diseases and disorders are on the rise.
Our assessment of the latest science leaves little room for
doubt; pesticides are one key driver of this sobering trend.

—October 2012 Report by Pesticide Action
Network North America (PANNA)

EAT ORGANIC FOODS!

The most important thing about food could be summarized in this way: eat God-made foods, not man-made foods. God-made foods are organic by design and heal us. GMO stands for "genetically modified organism," and GE stands for "genetically engineered." They are interchangeable terms. They are both man-altered foods. They pollute us with toxic chemicals.

In case you may not know, GMO crops have had their genetic DNA artificially altered. This is done by introducing genes from a totally different to make the plant super-resistant to pests or herbicides, thus creating a new set of genes. Then these engineered crops are also sprayed with millions of pounds of toxic chemicals every year!

GMOs came out in 1996 as the solution to world hunger. Many countries outside the U.S. banned synthetic manipulation of foods. They "opted" out. As of 2015, 38 countries have banned GMO crop cultivation. This includes 28 European countries, and Russia, Saudi Arabia, Germany, France, Norway, two African, and four South and Central American countries. More than 60 countries require foods to have GMO labeling. In contrast, the U.S. plants the most GMO crops of all countries, followed by Brazil, Argentina, Canada, and India. Together, these five countries make up 91% of the global GMO crops. More than half of the global GMO crops are soybeans followed by corn. In the U.S. and Canada, GMO food labeling is not required even though 64 countries around the world require it.

Why have so many countries banned GMOs? For health and environmental reasons. When you consume pesticides that are on the genetically modified foods, they accumulate in your body. Many studies show how the compounding effects of these genetically modified (GM) foods in a person's diet are negative and unhealthy. A study published in *Environmental Sciences Europe* shows that pesticides have been linked to cancer in laboratory animals. Rats fed GM corn showed severe liver and kidney damage as well as hormonal disruptions. No standardized methods to determine GMO safety have been established. This has worried world leaders and scientists, and should worry all of us. What harms lab animals is a danger in that it will harm humans as well. All of us carry some body burden of these GMO toxins and, many of us, unfortunately, suffer their cumulative effects.

In 2014, Irina Ermakova, VP of Russia's National Association for Genetic Safety said, "*It is necessary to ban GMOs… Methods of obtaining the GMOs are dangerous. Methods of obtaining the GMOs are not perfect; therefore, at this stage, all GMOs are dangerous. Consumption and use of*

GMOs obtained in such a way can lead to tumors, cancers and obesity among animals." The CDC noted that in children between ages 0 to 17, allergies jumped significantly from 1997–2001. They cannot say GMOs caused it; they simply established a link. The CDC, in 2015, also determined that the herbicide glyphosate, a key ingredient in farming pesticides, is "probably carcinogenic to humans." The U.S. EPA also reported that glyphosate caused DNA and chromosomal damage in human cells. GMOs have been linked to increased food allergens, internal organ damage, slowed brain growth, many gastrointestinal problems and headaches. Most disturbing, studies have linked low doses of these pesticides to increased risk of leukemia, breast cancer, prostate cancer, brain tumors, and lymphoma.

Children, fetuses, and pregnant women are most vulnerable. Pesticides pass from mother to baby in the womb and through breast milk. Children and fetuses with developing brains, bodies and immune systems are most greatly affected. This causes developmental delays, behavioral disorders, autism, and immune system damage leading to allergies and sensitivities.

"Organic" refers to the manner in which foods are raised. Organic foods are minimally processed and do not contain hormones, preservative chemicals, food colors, sweeteners or flavorings that were not originally in the food. Conventional, industrial-raised animals, not organic-raised animals, are fed an unnatural diet full of antibiotics, growth hormones, and animal byproducts. Organic foods are naturally superior in nutrition; they have powerful antioxidants, minerals, amino acids, enzymes and vitamins vital for hormone and body function. Reviews of multiple studies have shown that organic foods provide significantly greater amount of magnesium, vitamin C, iron, and much greater levels of antioxidant phytochemicals than their nonorganic counterparts. Organic fruits contain higher levels of flavonoids than GMO fruit and up to 50% more antioxidants. There are also significantly much lower levels of toxic chemicals such as nitrates and pesticide particles in organic foods.

In a study published in the British Journal of Nutrition in 2016, investigators analyzed 196 studies on milk and 67 studies on meat.

They found that the organic products had much higher levels of good fats and had many more essential minerals and antioxidants. They reported that the organic milk and meats had an astounding 50% more healthy omega-3 fatty acids and also less saturated fat, which is cardio-protective, neuro-protective and immune-protective. The organic milk also had 40% more conjugated linoleic acid and more iron, vitamin E and carotenoids.

Another study done by the same researchers and supported by the European Commission showed that organically grown crops had 60% more nutrients and antioxidants compared to nonorganic crops. The scientists put out a statement, saying, "*We have shown without doubt there are composition differences between organic and conventional food. These studies suggest that a switch to organic fruit, vegetables, meat and dairy products would provide significantly higher amounts of dietary antioxidants and omega-3 fatty acids.*" Based on another report in *British Journal of Nutrition*, scientists in Europe and the United States reviewed over 343 studies and concluded that organic crops and foods contained much higher concentrations of antioxidants than nonorganic foods.

We are what we eat; we do not want to be a vessel of toxic pesticides, chemicals and antibiotics. We have a choice every day. We need to eat organic food to get the antioxidants needed to build our immune system and sustain our body with complete nutrition. Be proactive. Eat organic Mother Nature foods. They are made to heal us and empower our immune systems.

CHAPTER 12

PowerHouse SuperFoods— Sustaining Health and Longevity

Tell me what you eat, I'll tell you who you are.

—Anthelme Brillat-Savarin,
1755–1826, famed epicure

EAT PLANT-BASED FOODS AS MUCH AS POSSIBLE!

Dietary antioxidants are powerful. They turn on or off the expression of thousands of genes. Foods and vitamins act as chemical signals that prepare the body for fighting disease and inflammation. They activate the immune system to defend against inflammation at the cellular level. Antioxidants are electron donors. Free radicals are electron takers that steal electrons in a cell membrane and denature the tissue or DNA. This is the beginning of inflammation, disease and cancer. We can fight this by eating abundant whole organic foods high in antioxidants.

Fresh organic fruits and vegetables have long been associated with extending the lifespan by protecting us from age-related diseases. Scientists have developed a method of measuring the antioxidant capacity of food. It's called ORAC, or oxygen radical antioxidant capacity. Generally, vegetables and fruits that are richer in color are usually rich in antioxidants. The deeper the color, the more phytochemicals they have. They are potent antioxidants that stimulate and protect the immune system and stimulate cancer cell destruction. The most nutrient-rich foods on the planet are leafy greens. Use tons of fresh herbs on everything because they are full of health-promoting nutrients, vitamins, minerals and pure antioxidants that fight inflammation.

POWERHOUSE SUPERFOODS

All our food calories, energy, come from three sources—carbohydrates, fats and proteins. Food nutrients have no calories and supply and support body functions. Examples of food nutrients include vitamins, minerals, fibers and phytochemicals. Below, I have listed PowerHouse Foods, rich in antioxidants.

Fiber-packed vegetables—artichokes, mushrooms, celery, Brussels sprouts, kale, spinach, sweet potatoes, yams, cauliflower, beets, cabbage, tomatoes, peppers, cucumbers, bok choy, garlic, leeks, asparagus, radish, broccoli, carrots, collard greens, seaweed, zucchini, eggplant, all leafy green lettuce, onions, broccoli, alfalfa, bean sprouts and sprouts of any kind.

Low-sugar, high-fiber fruit—avocados, apples, berries, lemons, limes, cherries, red grapes, kiwi, bananas, apricot, pears and oranges.

Wild-caught fatty fish and organic, grass-fed meat—cold water fish: salmon, cod, halibut, tuna, trout, haddock, sardines, shellfish (shrimp, crab, lobster, clams, oysters, mussels); organic, grass-fed meats: beef, chicken, turkey, duck, lamb, bison and pork, and pasture-raised organic eggs.

Fermented foods—kefir, miso, sauerkraut, apple cider vinegar, pickles, kimchi, Indian dosa or idlis, sourdough bread, organic yogurt, and kambucha.

Grains and beans—millet, quinoa, amaranth, buckwheat (a seed, not a grain), basmati rice, sorghum grain, lentils, mung and adzuki beans, organic soybean, flaxseed, chickpeas, white and black beans, and sprouted-grain bread.

Oils and fats from seeds, nuts and olives—fresh walnuts, Brazil nuts, pumpkin seeds, almonds, cashews, shelled peanuts, hazelnuts, pistachios, coconut oil, MCT oil, avocado oil, cold-pressed extra virgin olive oil, flaxseed oil, ghee, nut and seed butters, and pasture-fed butter.

PowerHouse spices and herbs—turmeric root and spice, cloves, cinnamon, cardamom, cayenne pepper, garlic, ginger, tamarind, fennel, basil, oregano, parsley, cilantro, ground peppercorn and Himalayan or Celtic salt.

PowerHouse drinks—alkaline "active" water, green tea, coconut water and kombucha

PowerHouse sweets—manuka honey, maple syrup and stevia

SUPERIOR BENEFITS OF GREEN TEA—ELIXIR OF LIFE!

Green tea is perhaps the healthiest and ultimate anti-aging beverage on the planet! A 5,000-year-old Chinese tradition that has spread to Japan and to the rest of the world. It is the drink most commonly enjoyed by centenarians around the world.

Green tea is a strong antioxidant, containing potent catechin polyphenols, which reduce systemic inflammation, protect DNA, protect and stimulate the immune system, increase higher tumor-killer cell rates and help prevent cancer metastasis. In some studies, the antioxidant potency of green tea was even more powerful than vitamin C or E. Green tea also has B vitamins, folate, manganese, potassium, magnesium and caffeine. It delays aging. As discussed previously, free radicals erode the body; however, antioxidant-rich green tea neutralizes the free radicals in the body. The powerful anti-oxidizing effect of its polyphenols can delay aging if you drink green tea regularly.

In human studies, green-tea drinkers had half the incidences of cancer as non-green tea drinkers. Green tea's catechin polyphenols neutralize the free radicals that cause premature aging and cancer and prevent the formation of carcinogens like nitrosamines. It limits cancer by restricting blood vessel growth and platelet adhesion. The antioxidant properties of green tea help weaken and kill cancer cells and strengthen normal cells. They induce autophagy and apoptotic cancer cell death, the body's cellular waste control process that defends the body from cancer and disease. In test-tube studies, green tea suppressed the tumor promoters in breast cancer.

Drinking green tea, without sugar, is best. Its alkaline nature and a powerful compound EGCG (epigallocatechin gallate) reduce appetite, increase metabolism, help improve fat-burning, help reduce the blood glucose levels, and help increase insulin release, preventing and controlling diabetes and abdominal obesity. A Japanese study found that those who drank the most green tea had a 42% lower risk of developing type 2 diabetes. Another study reviewing seven studies with 286,701 participants showed that green tea drinkers had an 18% lower risk of developing diabetes.

Green tea is also great for stress reduction. It contains L-theanine, an amino acid that easily crosses the blood—brain barrier to promote alpha brain waves to induce calmness, so you feel relaxed yet alert without drowsiness. Studies show theanine also enhances the brain's ability to learn and focus better and, for centuries, it has been used by monks to help in meditation. One study showed green tea drinkers were 44% less likely to suffer from depressive symptoms.

Heart disease is the number one killer in the U.S.; green tea pro-longs life by preventing heart attacks and promoting heart heath. The antioxidants in green tea reduce blood pressure and improve cardiac health by expanding the arterial lining, thus improving blood flow and preventing arterial blood clots that eventually cause heart attacks. Green tea polyphenolic compounds increase the antioxidant capacity of the blood, protecting LDL particle oxidation and lowering LDL cholesterol, triglyceride and total cholesterol levels.

The Ohsaki National Health Insurance Cohort Study is one of the largest studies ever conducted. It followed 40,530 Japanese adults for 11 years. The subjects that drank five or more cups of green tea a day were 16% (23% lower in women, 12% lower in men) less likely to die from all causes than those who drank less than one cup a day. Green tea drinkers were 26% (31% in women, 22% in men) less likely to die from heart disease and 36% (42% in women, 35% in men) less likely to die from strokes. The lead researcher, Shinichi Kuriyama, said, *"The most important finding is that green tea may prolong people's lives through reducing the risk of cardiovascular disease."* Another study conducted showed green tea drinkers had up to a 31% lower risk of heart disease.

Green tea may help fight Alzheimer's and Parkinson's diseases and memory loss. Japanese researchers have shown that the powerful catechin polyphenols of green tea reduce damage from free radical in rats' brains. The rats with green tea had much less memory loss and fewer beta-amyloid protein plaque, which is found in brains suffering from Alzheimer's disease.

Green tea has also been shown to prevent tooth decay. It is a natural, safe source of fluoride. Fluoride helps our teeth be resistant to acids. The tea components have been found to destroy viruses and bacteria of the teeth and throat and prevent dental cavities and bad breath.

Green tea drinkers in general don't get as sick as non-green tea drinkers due to the immune-boosting benefits. Tea contains antigens that help prevent bacterial and viral infections.

Dr. Carrie Ruxton, a public health nutritionist from Kings College London, and her colleagues say tea is even better for you than water, *"Drinking tea is actually better for you than drinking water. Water is essentially replacing fluid. Tea replaces fluids and contains antioxidants, so it's got two things going for it."*

BENEFITS OF APPLE CIDER VINEGAR (ACV)

Organic unfiltered apple cider vinegar (ACV) has several medical benefits. Its main active ingredient is acetic acid, and it also contains friendly bacteria, enzymes, proteins and some antioxidants. ACV is a natural probiotic, replacing the gut flora with friendly bacteria, and it alkalizes the body's pH. Even though this is an acidic product, it goes through "an alkaline tide" through salivary digestive enzymes, turning it alkaline. This helps prevent disease; just by balancing gut flora, we increase our immune system's potential. Numerous studies have shown ACV shrinks or kills cancer cells in lab rats and isolated cells in test tubes.

ACV also kills bad bacteria; it has been used to preserve food for centuries. It has been shown to inhibit E. coli growth, which causes food poisoning.

Multiple studies have shown how ACV is great to lower blood sugars and improve insulin sensitivity, thus greatly benefiting type 2 diabetic patients. Studies have shown drinking ACV after a high-carb meal can help reduce blood sugars as much as 34%.

I recommend drinking 1 to 2 teaspoons of ACV, straight or diluted in 12 ounces of warm water, to start off. Increase slowly to 1 to 2 table-spoons, then to twice a day, as tolerated. Use freely in soups, and spray onto salads.

BENEFITS OF MANUKA HONEY

Manuka honey is produced from New Zealand bees. It is one of the most sought out and beneficial forms of honey in the world. The Maori, the native people of New Zealand, have been using manuka honey for generations for its amazing healing purposes. It is their "go-to medicine." It is an anti-oxidant, anti-bacterial and anti-inflammatory PowerFood. This honey has powerful, natural health benefits along with tasting absolutely decadent, rich in flavor. It is four times more potent in immune-boosting nutrients than other honeys and contains B vitamins, amino acids, iron, copper, magnesium, zinc and others. It is rated by UMF (Unique Manuka Factor) trademark standards, determined by anti-bacterial properties of the honey at the time of packaging. Higher UMF ratings mean stronger antibacterial properties. The higher the UMF, the pricier the honey. I recommend a UMF of 16 to get the full benefits of manuka honey. It should be labeled as such in front of the container. It is absolutely worth every delicious drop! It's a pure, organic and time-tested superfood!

1. Anti-Bacterial Properties—Manuka honey has powerful, natural high antibacterial levels. It kills bacteria that cause strep throat, cold sores, skin infections, stomach ulcers and sore throats. It is effective as a dressing to heal skin cuts, wounds, burns and ulcers when applied externally.

Even more impressive is that research shows that along with other medications, manuka honey fights off staph infections (MRSA), the drug-resistant superbugs that usually traditionally require mega-antibiotics to treat. Studies also show manuka honey helps treat and prevent gum disease, gingivitis and periodontal disease. Periodontal disease has been directly connected to heart disease. Healthy teeth and gums keep a healthy heart. Studies from the University of Otago, School of Dentistry in New Zealand, show that sucking or chewing on manuka honey products decreased plaque by 35% and decreased bleeding gums in gingivitis patients by 35%. So far, there has been no antibiotic resistance to manuka honey.

2. Allergy and Sinus Relief—Manuka honey is full of high pollen content and can desensitize your body to other pollens. Studies show that it helps treat and reduce symptoms of allergies and sinus symptoms. Taking a teaspoon regularly reduces symptoms during the allergy season.

3. Acts as a Probiotic—It soothes the gut lining and nurtures good bacterial growth. Therefore, it acts as an immune booster and helps fight off bad bacteria and viruses. It helps digestion and helps take away bloating and gas, heartburn, upset stomach, colonic pain and IBS pain, and soothes gastric ulcers.

4. Sleep—Manuka honey before bedtime helps release melatonin into the brain, a natural sleeping aid to help have deeper sleep.

5. Great skin—It's a great natural moisturizer that heals, hydrates and brightens skin, and improves skin tone with its intense succulent antioxidants. It puts a layer of moisture on the skin to kill off free radicals and heal scars and acne. It works great as a mask; apply directly to the skin, leave it on for 15 minutes (or an hour to get better results) and rinse off. It also treats dry, itchy skin that is eczema-prone by keeping in moisture and reducing inflammation.

Be cautious if you have a honey allergy; consult your doctor first if you are unsure or have any adverse or questionable reaction after exposure to honey. I recommend stirring one teaspoon of manuka honey into your green tea, yogurt, fruit, or sprouted grain toast. You can also apply it directly on your skin and take by mouth directly.

SUPERIOR BENEFIT OF NUTS

Considering you don't have a nut allergy, try to eat at least 2 to 3 handfuls of nuts every day. Nuts are a powerful source of vegetable proteins. An Adventist Health Study (AHS) reported people who ate two ounces of nuts, five days a week, lived an average of two years longer and also had half the heart disease risk as their counterparts who didn't eat nuts. Nuts are full of soluble fiber and monounsaturated fats, lowering bad cholesterol (LDL) and raising good cholesterol (HDL), thereby lowering heart disease. Eat whatever nuts and seeds you enjoy, about 2 to 3 handfuls a day.

Soaking nuts overnight and sprouting them is one of the healthiest ways to eat nuts. They are much easier to digest and absorb in the gut, allowing greater absorption of minerals and trace elements.

Grains, such as lentils and legumes, should also be eaten sprouted. Soak them overnight to allow them to be more easily digestible and absorbable. Whole grains not sprouted contain toxins that irritate the gut flora and can inhibit digestive enzymes and cause gas and bloating. Many people don't eat beans and lentils because of this reason; try soaking the legumes overnight in water with a splash of apple cider vinegar. The sprouted grains will digest better and not cause gut discomfort.

CHAPTER 13

Water! Water! Water!

Life is not merely being alive but being well.

—Marcus Valerius Martialis

IT IS ESTIMATED THAT 75% OF AMERICANS ARE CHRONICALLY dehydrated. The body is composed of 70% water. Amazingly, we were designed in sync with Mother Earth, which is about 71% water. Water preserves life. Our blood is composed of about 80% water, our muscles are about 70% water and our brain cells 85%.

The majority of people are walking around chronically dehydrated, tired and have poor memory. Water not only brings nutrients to the body's tissue, it also helps flush out toxins. The problem is that people don't drink enough water and, when they do, it's poor quality and doesn't even absorb properly to gain its benefits. Ninety-five percent of water is absorbed in the small intestine. Thus, everything comes back to gut health. Maintaining good gut health is critical for proper hydration.

Most water that people drink is "dead" or "lifeless" water. It comes from bottled or tap water, which has gone through basic filtration, having low osmolality. Osmolality measures the concentration of particles like glucose and sodium, which helps the water get to the body effectively through the small intestine, where the majority of water is absorbed. Water that has been pumped or piped, and then sits in plastic for months is chaotic at the molecular level and doesn't penetrate into the body's cells. For water to easily penetrate at the cellular level, it needs to have an electrolyte balance. This optimizes water osmolality. This is termed energetically "active" or "live" water.

Research has suggested that we can easily super-charge our water and prevent chronic dehydration by just adding salt, spices and fruit. This is something everyone can do easily. Add a tiny pinch of Himalayan sea salt to daily water. I recommend reverse osmotic water with added minerals from a pinch of Himalayan sea salt.

Remember, we were born of water and salt. We were all carried in the womb, full of amniotic water, a form of saline solution or salt water, a perfect electrolyte balance of "active" water for nine months. It sustained our life. When we were delivered into the world from the womb, we entered a symbiotic world full of salt water because the earth is made up of 71% water. Our body cries, sweats and urinates electrolytes. We must replenish with "active" electrolyte water to sustain our best innate fighting powers and balance.

HIMALAYAN SEA SALT

Himalayan sea salt is a soft pink unrefined salt crystal, rich in 84 essential minerals, such as sodium, iodine, zinc, magnesium, iron and potassium. You can barely taste any difference with just a pinch in a liter of water. This satisfies your thirst, keeps the body at the cellular level well-hydrated and replenishes the body with much needed minerals. This is a simple way to create natural, super-charged "active" electrolyte water.

Both Celtic and Himalayan salts have 84 trace minerals. Both are powerful, natural ways to super-charge our water quality. Himalayan sea salt has been matured over 250 million years and used for healing in old traditions, especially Tibetan and Ayurvedic traditions. It not only super-hydrates the body; it also detoxes the body by pH balancing it, decreases cramps and promotes thyroid, adrenal, kidney and gall-bladder health, as well as the health of the sinuses. It supports hormone and sugar balance too. Both salts are known to have antimicrobial- and antibacterial-promoting properties that help naturally purify water from invisible-to-the-eye bugs.

There are other great medical benefits to the salts. Since the 1800s, Europeans have visited salt mines to breathe salt-rich air. Ancient salt mines from Austria and Germany, famously called "white gold" mines, have had centuries of healing effects on its visitors. When the salt air is inhaled, it passes through the entire respiratory system, so its antimicrobial properties detox and purify the lungs and sinus fields. The benefits include improved asthma, allergies, eczema and lung function and, for many, it reduces or eliminates snoring. The inhaled salts also help with deep relaxation and stress relief. What's more, the inhaled minerals aid in digestion, bowel movement and gut flora balance. To get these benefits at home, I suggest getting a Himalayan salt inhaler. I also strongly recommend using a neti pot with Himalayan salts and distilled water to get the same sinus and respiratory benefits.

Himalayan sea salts in a bath are a great detox too. From Iceland, England, Hungary, Italy, Germany, Greece, France and Spain, there are geothermal salt baths, pools, therapeutic waterfalls and springs that have been used for centuries for such whole-body healing purposes. Using a handful of sea salts in a bath draws out toxins and deep cleanses the skin. The minerals are also excellent to ease joint pain, allergies, muscle aches, arthritis, stress release and the induction of deep relaxation.

HOW MUCH WATER SHOULD I DRINK?

To stay well-hydrated, drink half your body weight, in ounces. Daily. If you get bored with water, add a squeeze of fresh lemon, lime, cucumber slices, aloe, orange, mint or basil leaf to your water. The vitamins and fiber in the water balance the body's pH and make the tonic water "active."

The best way to start your day should be with drinking eight ounces of hot water with a squeeze of lemon and a dash of cayenne pepper. This is an age-old Ayurvedic cleansing ritual. Try to start your day with this powerful hydrating cleanse.

Drinking green tea is another great way to stay hydrated, as long as no sugar is added. It's alkaline, full of powerful antioxidants, and easily gets absorbed.

Most organic fruits and vegetables are about 70% water, packed with phytonutrients and fiber. Some of best hydrating fruits or vegetables are apples, citrus, cherries, pears, plums, berries, watermelon, avocados, all leafy greens, onions, asparagus, cauliflower, cabbage, celery, cucumbers, broccoli and carrots.

Try to avoid regular table salt as it has been heavily processed, bleached and stripped of minerals, and is full of additives as well. Regular table salt raises blood pressure, increases thirst and bloating, and taxes the kidneys to work extra hard to filter and excrete the sodium.

Avoid tap water; it may contain contaminants and harmful chemicals. I suggest using a water filter that does alkalinizing or ionizing, and a carbon filter to remove chemicals, heavy metals, and pathogens.

CHAPTER 14

Vegetarian vs. Non-Vegetarian Eating

The fate of a nation depends on the way that they eat.
— Anthelme Brillat-Savarin,
1755–1826, famed epicure

MANY PEOPLE THINK THAT YOU HAVE TO EAT ANIMAL proteins to get all the essential amino acids needed and that plant proteins are incomplete. Not true—plant proteins can provide a complete array of essential amino acids. Research has shown unrefined plant foods supply the greatest protection against developing cancer and disease.

High fat animal-derived foods (meat, dairy, milk, cheese, butter) have repeatedly been connected with cancer. Studies show that men and women who ate meat every day or had butter and cheese 3 to 4 times a week, are 3 to 4 times as likely to develop breast cancer and prostate cancer as those who seldom ate meat or not at all.

ANIMAL VS. PLANT PROTEINS

Animal proteins—increase bad cholesterol, increase cancer risk, promote cancer growth, promote bone loss and accelerate aging due to high saturated fats and low fiber.

Plant proteins—lower bad cholesterol, are a cancer protector and preventer, promote bone strength, and decrease aging due to phyto-chemicals, antioxidants and high fiber.

You don't have to become a vegan or vegetarian. Most of these studies were probably conducted on non-organic processed meats. Most studies don't detail if the meats used in the studies were GMO, processed or organic. It is absolutely important to give up hormone- and GMO-filled meats, eggs and animal proteins, and convert fully to organic, grass-fed beef and meats if you truly enjoy your meats.

The Mediterranean and Okinawa diets both contain meat—just clean, limited levels of it. In fact, the Okinawa tradition loves pork. They roast the pig in celebration of life and fully enjoy every part of it. The Mediterranean diet consists of meat also, just in limited amounts.

If you have a strong family history or previous medical history of high cholesterol or cardiac disease, or you have had a heart attack, then perhaps you should consider becoming a vegetarian. Try to give up 80% of meat and animal proteins like cheese. This means eating meat once a week (or less). Eat more wild fish, lentils, organic tofu, eggs, nuts, nutrient-rich leafy greens and fruits.

I generally recommend to my patients that they eat grass-fed organic meat and meat-based foods, such as cheese, minimally—only 1 to 2 times a week. Meat restriction is important, not meat elimina-tion. Quality of the meat is paramount; do grass-fed, organic meat as much as possible. I recommend eating more wild-caught fish, wild-caught seafood and pasture-raised, organic eggs. Meat should be a side dish, alongside seasonal vegetables.

Exciting new evidence has been surfacing that shows that organic, grass-fed beef, unlike its GMO counterpart, is packed with good omega-3 fats, antioxidants and conjugated linoleic acid, a type of fat associated with a reduced risk of high cholesterol, cancer and heart disease.

CHEW YOUR FOOD AND EAT SLOWLY!

Fear less, hope more; eat less, chew more; whine less, breathe more; talk less, say more; hate less, love more; and all the good things will be yours.

—Swedish Proverb

We do not have teeth in our gut. We must eat slowly and chew properly. The process of chewing food breaks down food into a pulp, so we can absorb the nutrients in the gut. Otherwise, the nutritious food you eat has limited benefits because the digestive enzymes in the gut cannot break down bulky, chunky food pieces.

Studies show that normal weight people chew more slowly than their overweight and obese counterparts. Numerous studies have concluded eating more slowly leads to feeling fuller, i.e., satiety. We have an indigenous appetite-regulating hormone—leptin—that tells our body when we are full and to stop eating. These hormones need time to feel the stretch receptors in the stomach and to signal the brain to stop eating. If we eat too fast, we can overeat before these hormones have time to signal us to stop. This is when eating becomes a mindless, endless hobby. In a British 2008 study, eating quickly and eating until full triples a person's risk of becoming overweight.

How slowly do you have to eat? Scientists report that it takes about 15 to 20 minutes to signal your brain feelings of fullness. So, eat more slowly, chew well, taste and enjoy your food!

INTERMITTENT FASTING

The best of all medicines are resting and fasting.

—Benjamin Franklin

Try to stop eating by 6 PM. It is best to stop eating 3 to 4 hours before your bedtime to allow food to pass through the stomach and start digesting. This allows you to fast through the night for at least 12 to 16 hours. Intermittent fasting is more of a time-restricted eating plan. You eat your calories during the day hours and fast during the sleeping hours. Most people tend to eat late and eat their biggest meal at night, causing gut issues, weight gain, heartburn and insulin resistance, which causes type 2 diabetes.

There is strong scientific research suggesting fasting lowers body fat, increases insulin sensitivity and reduces inflammation. When we fast, we put our cells under stress, challenging them in a good way so that they strengthen and become more resistant to disease.

PART III

LIFESTYLE

CHAPTER 15

Exercise Maxes Out Mitochondria

*Lack of activity destroys the good condition of every
human being, while movement and methodical
physical exercise save it and preserve it.*

—Plato

RESEARCH OVERWHELMINGLY SUPPORTS THAT EXERCISE significantly reduces cancer risk. Studies show that up to 40% of Americans will develop cancer. In contrast, only 14% of active, regular-exercising Americans will develop cancer. Evidence supports that exercising 30 minutes, four times a week reduces breast cancer risk by 75%.

A study in Norway involving more than 25,000 women between the ages of 20 and 54 studied the correlation of regular exercise and risk of breast cancer. The results were that younger, premenopausal women (under 45 years old) who exercised regularly had a 62% less risk than sedentary women. The risk reduction was highest for lean females who exercised more than four hours per week; these women had a 72% reduction in breast cancer risk.

As previously discussed, fat cells can convert testosterone and DHEA into the harmful estrogen, E1, in both men and women, increasing risks for cancer and heart disease. When you exercise regularly, you lose fat and also lose one of your body's main sources of potentially harmful estrogens.

Another study from the Health Survey for England and the Scottish Health Survey assessed data of 80,306 adults over a 14-year span. The study showed that adults who did strength training reduced their risk of premature death from any cause by 23% and reduced the risk of overall cancer death by 31%.

Data shows those who exercise regularly also have a higher sex drive and enhanced orgasms. Working out helps improve self-confidence, sexual functioning and satisfaction. A study reported that 60-year olds who exercised regularly had the same amount of sex and sexual pleasure as those decades younger. Regular exercising keeps you sexually hungry and confident. Exercise and sex regenerate the brain with endorphins, a natural "happy" charge.

Regular exercise also promotes gut healing. As discussed in an earlier chapter, a recent study from San Francisco State University showed that cardiovascular exercise can boost gut health by increasing the good bacteria in the gut's microbiome. In the study, students who worked out on a treadmill were compared to those who didn't. Also subjects had food logs, stool samples, and had their gut bacteria analyzed. Those students with higher fitness levels had higher levels of firmicutes bacteris, a healthy gut bacterium that prevents leaky gut syndrome. Lead researcher, Ryan Durk, reported, *"We now know that exercise is crucial for increasing beneficial bacteria in the gut."*

Benefits of regular exercise include the prevention of memory loss and the sharpening of memory. It also reduces cortisol levels, which means it reduces and helps manage chronic and acute stress.

According to Dr. Mark Tarnopolsky, a professor and expert researcher on mitochondria, less than 20% of people workout optimally, that is 150 minutes per week, or about 20 minutes per day. Doing cardio, interval training, or high intensity training, along with resistance training, are all great exercise routines. Doing cardio twice a week, weight training twice a week or combining them—so working out four times a week—is excellent. According to Dr. Tarnopolsky, both cardio and resistance training have been shown to increase mitochondrial production.

Mitochondria are the cells' power centers and are important in cell regeneration and repair. The more mitochondria, the more efficient the mitochondria, and the better each cell works to generate energy and repair itself. As discussed previously, scientists have discovered that destroyed mitochondria equal increased cell death, which leads to disease and cancer.

The key to regenerating mitochondria is maxing out during cardio exercise, thus making them super-efficient. Dr. Tarnopolsky says that endurance exercises can double the amount of mitochondria in your muscles. Cardio or endurance exercise, such as cycling twice a week for 30 to 45 minutes and walking once a week for three months, doubles the mitochondria and increases skin collagen production, both of which are "youthening" effects.

His data also found that routine exercise increases levels of a molecule that protects telomeres. Telomeres are protective caps on chromosomes, and routine exercises prevents their shortening. The longer the telomeres, the longer the lifespan. Dr. Tarnopolsky showed even in older adults, resistance training three times a week increased their mitochondria by 30%. Dr. Tarnopolsky's research proves that exercise restores and improves mitochondria function and slows down aging at a cellular and telomere level. He suggests that by exercising regularly, you can slow down your speed of aging and can increase your lifespan by five years.

ADDED BENEFITS OF RESISTANCE TRAINING

Those who do not find time for exercise will have to find time for illness.

—Edward Smith-Stanley,
three-time Prime Minister of the U.K.

Following are additional benefits of resistance training:

1. Increases testosterone, estrogen and HGH production
2. Lowers circulation of bad estrogens and restores a healthy estrogen and testosterone balance

3. Burns fat efficiently

4. Improves bone density, reducing osteoporosis risk

5. Improves flexibility or joint pain

6. Prevents sarcopenia (muscle weakness)

7. Improves insulin sensitivity in muscle tissue, preventing type 2 diabetes

8. Increases cellular mitochondria

9. Improves collagen production for better skin

10. Revs up confidence and sex drive

Bank your good health, especially with regular exercise, to get you through challenging times. Life is dynamic and unpredictable, so take each day as a blessing and do your best to bank good habits.

Regular exercise should never be compromised, especially during high stress times or on vacations. Vacation is a great time to go walking on the beach or go by foot to dinner or exploring. When people are faced with a crisis or heavy stress, they tend to abandon their workouts. Working out in times of heavy stress helps you cope. That is the most critical time to not give up regular exercise. Do your best to keep your good habits in times of heavy stress or distress. The endorphins will help you cope and recover through the pain.

In times of tragedy or crisis, we feel immobilized with pain. It is important to realize that sleep and time heals us. So be kind to yourself and try to go for walks. Being your best and eating healthy, working out regularly, taking vitamins and balancing your hormones will help you get through the most difficult times with a net of sustained health below you. Your banked good habits will sustain your recovery and help you cope during times of deep crisis. Exercise is a physical transformation that can empower you to ultimately become the best version of yourself!

CHAPTER 16

Sleep Restores
the Immune System

O sleep, O gentle Sleep, Nature's soft nurse.
—William Shakespeare

SLEEP REGENERATES THE SKIN, BODY AND BRAIN. Unfortunately, many people do not value their sleep and sacrifice their sleep to working, watching mindless TV, browsing the internet or some other activity. Sleep is vital for youth and health preservation and life extension.

The CDC reports that more than one-third of Americans consistently do not get enough sleep. This increases their risk of chronic disease and cognitive decline. Studies have shown that sleeping six or less hours a night increases the risk of diabetes, depression, anxiety, obesity, memory loss and heart disease.

Sleep deprivation produces the bad hormone cortisol. The body perceives the lack of sleep as stress and responds by producing the stress chemical, cortisol. A University of Chicago study analyzed healthy college men who were kept up until 1 AM for nearly six nights and then awakened at 5 AM. After six nights of sleep deprivation with only four hours of sleep per night, all these 20-year-olds had cortisol levels of 60-year-old men!

Cortisol, the fight-or-flight hormone, is responsible for abdominal weight gain, insulin resistance or diabetes, anxiety, higher cholesterol and food cravings. Another study monitored 70,000 nurses, who slept only 5 to 7 hours per night. They had significantly more heart attacks than their counterparts who slept eight hours per night.

Dr. Rebecca Robbins, sleep expert and researcher, explains, "*During a good night's rest, your body works to remove dead blood cells and dead brain cells, and clears the pathways for new synapses to take place so that new blood and brain cells can replace old ones.*" She also reported that the brain gets rid of 60% more toxins when you get the proper amount of sleep.

CRITICAL BENEFITS OF SLEEP (7 TO 8 HOURS/NIGHT)

Sleep is the best meditation.

—Dalai Lama

1. Increases brain function, focus and memory processing. Studies have found a direct link between sleep, productivity and intelligence. It is during sleep that the brain processes new information, stores memory and recharges and strengthens neuronal connections.

2. Increases weight loss because leptin is released during sleep. Leptin, the "full" hormone, regulates appetite control. Lack of sleep increases ghrelin, the "hunger" hormone, which makes you crave more food and just pleasure eat. Leptin opposes ghrelin, suppressing hunger and helping to prevent overeating. Sleep increases leptin levels, which means less hunger, less eating and less obesity.

3. Decreases cortisol in body, which helps improve stress, anxiety and depression.

4. Increases testosterone production in men and estrogen production in females. HGH (human growth hormone), the ultimate anti-aging hormone, is produced during deep sleep.

5. Increases the immune system's cell recovery. It increases production of NK cells (natural killer cells), your innate defenses against cancer, bacteria and viruses.

6. Decreases rate of skin and hair aging by increasing estrogen, testosterone and growth hormone, which prevents wrinkles and loose skin, and helps grow hair and tighten, brighten and hydrate skin. Testosterone for men increases skin quality, tone and hair growth.

7. Increases sex drive, just by producing more sex hormones during deep sleep.

CHAPTER 17

Detoxing Preserves the Body

The doctor of the future will give no medicine
but will interest his patients in the care of the human frame,
in diet and in the cause and prevention of disease.

—Thomas Edison

TOXINS LOWER OUR INNATE IMMUNE SYSTEM'S ABILITIES AND damage our DNA. Daily toxins are water, plastics, air, GMO foods, diets full of beef, milk, sugar and alcohol, drugs, tobacco and toxins in daily cleaners and makeup. It is exceedingly important to protect yourself from and limit exposure to toxins, and to detox regularly.

Detoxing includes fixing gut health, exercising, adequately hydrating, properly breathing, being hormonally balanced, taking vitamins to detox liver and the rest of the body, eating pH-balanced foods like vegetables and other plant-based foods, taking probiotics and cutting out sugars, processed foods, GMO foods, and toxic household products and cosmetics.

We all accumulate environmental and industrial chemical burdens every day. Unfortunately, in the U.S., cosmetics, lotions and hair and body products are not tested for toxicology and safety. Cosmetic products and ingredients are only vetted for color additives. Products used every day, like makeup, hair care products, deodorants, skin care products, lotions, fragrances, perfumes and toothpaste, have chemicals like parabens and phthalates. These chemicals disrupt our hormones.

Parabens are chemicals that mimic estrogen and interfere with body mechanisms. In animal studies, these "estrogen mimickers" or xenoestrogens, are linked to cancers, infertility, obesity, and organ interference, and especially thyroid function.

Natural estrogen is good for us; however, xenoestrogens are not. They are "estrogen-like" chemicals and toxins associated with cancers and disease because they disrupt proper hormonal balance; in par-ticular, estrogen. They bind to the body's estrogen receptors and can trigger abnormal processes.

A scientific study shows that an average American woman exposes herself to 168 personal care chemicals and products daily. Teenage females on average use 217! All these chemicals have a toxic burden on the body, altering the body's hormonal chemistry over time.

Use the Skin Deep Cosmetic Database from the Environmental Working Guide (EWG) to research your cosmetics and how safe they truly are for your body.

Avoid food and water in plastic bottles and wrapping of all kind. Plastic bottles leach plasticizer chemicals called phthalates into the water when exposed to heat or are bottled too long. Phthalates dis-rupt and interfere with the production of sex hormones. They are in household cleaning products, food packaging, fragrances, cosmetics, and personal care products. They are chemicals used as binding agents and to also make plastics more flexible. Other plastic wraps have chemicals like PVC, polyvinyl chloride, which is a known car-cinogen, that also disrupts hormonal balance and is connected to infertility, obesity and tissue and organ damage.

It is critical to consider "timing of exposure" to chemical toxins, especially for pregnant women. Prenatal development and puberty are when the body's cells are developing rapidly, so the organs are highly vulnerable. Pregnant women should avoid chemical-laden personal care products as much as possible; they are hormone disruptors. On CBS's *60 Minutes*, Lesley Stahl reported that the higher the level of phthalates in the mother's urine during pregnancy, the greater occurrence of problems in young boys. Stahl commented that *"phthalates may be causing a slow and steady de-masculinization of men."* Phthalate exposure has been linked to early puberty in girls, which also is an increased risk factor for later-life breast cancer.

The European Union (E.U.), 28 countries, and Canada are much stricter on their cosmetic regulations than the U.S. The E.U. is strict and prohibits in cosmetics the use of hazard-based chemicals linked to cancer and birth defects. The E.U. adopted strict laws in 2003 and enforces them, banning 1,328 chemicals from cosmetics that are known or suspected to cause cancer, fertility problems, genetic mutations or birth defects. In contrast, the U.S. FDA has only banned 11 chemicals from cosmetics. The E.U. law requires heavy vetting and mandatory testing of all cosmetics. The U.S. needs to adopt such strict regulations and vetting of cosmetic toxins to protect its people from unnecessary hazardous chemicals and toxic burdens that disrupt hormones.

WHAT CAN WE DO FOR DAILY DETOXING?

Being aware of such toxins and avoiding them much as possible is most important. This is called proactive prevention. Next, if we are exposed daily, we must adopt daily detoxing methods to prevent toxic accumulation and burden.

The single most important factor in detoxing starts with adequate hydration. That means drinking half your body weight in ounces daily. Into your water squeeze fresh lemon, add a pinch of cayenne pepper or Himalayan sea salt, or both as both aid in gentle detoxing. Drink out of glass or stainless-steel containers.

Drinking green tea is a great way to detox every day. As discussed earlier, green tea is a powerful detoxing tonic!

Take powerful supplements full of antioxidants. I discuss them in detail in the next chapter: curcumin, vitamin D3, ALA, omega-3 fish oils, probiotics, S-acytle glutathione, resveratrol and system enzymes.

Avoid plastic storage; use glass containers. In general, avoid plastic-wrapped foods. When buying plastic, use recycling codes 1, 2 or 5 because they don't contain phthalates. Avoid non-stick cooking pans. Buy fragrance-free products, especially shampoo and conditioner. Buy products that say "phthalate-free" or "DEP-free."

Chlorella is a great detoxing supplement you can take every day. It is a single-celled alga packed with proteins, chlorophyll, fatty acids, vitamins and minerals. It detoxifies mercury, lead and dioxin.

Infrared saunas help detox fat cells. They are different from typical saunas in that they remove 7 to 8 times more pollutants. They increase blood flow and cellular repair. Taking chlorella, 2–3 grams, before the sauna treatment helps release more toxins. Also, using a loofa or dry brush for lymphatic stimulation drives out more toxins too. Using it for 20 minutes, 4 to 5 times a week, helps detox the body.

Get detoxing houseplants. Research shows that certain house-plants have air-purifying effects. According to the Environmental Protection Agency (EPA), indoor air quality is in the top five risks to public health. This is due to home materials made with toxic chemi-cals such as vinyl flooring, carpets and air fresheners.

On the next page are listed some of the best houseplants to remove chemicals from cleaning products, carpets, flooring, plastics, paints, airborne gases and particles, and formaldehyde. And, in turn, these plants pump out fresh oxygen. NASA (National Aeronautics and Space Administration) put out a list of houseplants that improve indoor air pollutants, such as cigarette smoke, organic solvents and possibly radon. This is a list of detoxing houseplants that you should place throughout your home and office.

THE BEST HOUSEPLANTS

Following is a list of the best houseplants to help you detox your environment.

- Devil's ivy
- Purple waffle plant
- Aloe vera
- Mother-in-law's tongue
- Peace lily
- Rubber plant
- English Ivy
- Ficus
- Gerbera daisies
- Areca palm
- Money plant
- Red-edged dracaena

Losing bad fat by regular exercise is a great detox. Fat stores toxins from alcohol, marijuana, cigarettes and previously-used prescriptive drugs. Exercising burns off bad fat cells and releases the toxins stored in the bad fat cells. We previously discussed how fat cells can convert to estrogen, directly posing a higher risk of cancer, for both men and women. Routine exercise is a great detox because you sweat out the toxins, literally. Make it a habit to work out four times a week to burn off fat and toxins.

Remember, you have a choice every day to be healthier—or to be sicker. Being proactive and mindful of what you put on your skin, in your mouth, or in the air you breathe, all matters for hormonal balance and life extension.

CHAPTER 18

Nutritional Supplements to Maximize Wellness

I believe that you can, by taking some simple and inexpensive measures, lead a longer life and extend your years of well-being. My most important recommendation is that you take vitamins every day in optimum amounts to supplement the vitamins that you receive in your food.

—Linus Pauling, PhD,
two-time Nobel Prize Laureate

TAKING QUALITY VITAMINS IS ESSENTIAL FOR LIFE EXTENSION and reducing risks of chronic disease and cancer. High-grade medical vitamins are antioxidants and anti-inflammatory powerhouses for bolstering the immune system, rejuvenating and transforming the entire body, and sustaining vibrant health and longevity.

It is important we realize that every day we have a CHOICE to empower our body with innate immunity to defend against cancer and disease. We are exposed daily to stress and toxins. The body has so much to do and process to keep it balanced and prevent inflammation. Eating organic and plant-based foods as much as possible, calorie restriction, sleeping seven hours, exercising four times a week and coping with stress in a healthy way all make a huge difference to increase our own "heavy guns," or innate immune system, to fight for us. Combining these powerful anti-aging habits with taking superior quality supplements super-charges the immune system and lengthens the lifespan.

We have to arm the immune system with antioxidant power to fight daily aging and oxidation stress. Remember, oxidation stress and free radicals are damaging to the body. Antioxidants quench free radicals, protect us from oxidative damage, activate the cells' own internal fighting powers and win the battle of disease for the body. The more antioxidants we can consume, the greater our resistance to inflammation and disease formation. It is critical to eat more antioxidant power-packed fruits and vegetables and take superior supplements. Inflammation is fire in the body. The antioxidants put out the fire, so load up!

WHAT IS AUTOPHAGY?

Autophagy is the body's natural way of detoxing and eliminating cellular wastes. It is the "clean-up" process the cells do by themselves to prevent disease and cancer. It's a highly regulated process to recycle damaged and dysfunctional cells. This process also specifically happens in the mitochondria and is called mitophagy. It both degrades and replaces cellular debris, the hallmark of preventing disease and cancer. There is also a process, apoptosis or programmed cell death, that acts to keep cells in a state of homeostasis.

A diet full of fresh fruits and vegetables, along with daily high-quality nutritional supplements up-regulates autophagy and activates apoptosis of unhealthy cells.

What Are Some Super Vitamins That Increase Autophagy?

- Vitamin D3
- Curcumin
- Green tea polyphenol (EGCG)
- Resveratrol
- ALA
- NAC
- NAD+

Supplementation is necessary. In an ideal world without GMOs, environmental and water toxins, we could act otherwise. Medical-grade supplements "super-charge" the immune system, preserve and regenerate stem cells, gently detox the body daily and support brain, heart and gut health. I am suggesting supplementation only after first getting most of our vitamins and minerals from whole organic food sources.

Here is a summary of superior supplements, which I highly recommend to super-charge the immune system and extend the lifespan. Take a superior multivitamin along with the following vitamins (given below). Please consult your functional medicine doctor to help tailor dosing and determine the ones best for you. Remember, less is more when optimizing your nutrition and exercise.

Throughout my book, I refer frequently to these supplements because they are interconnected to hormone balance, health preservation and cancer prevention. It is so exciting that, along with restoring hormones, eating right, sleeping, exercising and taking supplements, we can extend our lifespans and rev up our own immune defenses!

Note: I'm sharing my generally recommended dosages here but please work with your healthcare provider to make sure you take the right dosages of all supplements for you and your body.

POWERFUL NUTRACEUTICALS

Resveratrol (more details in Chapter 18)

- Mimics the effects of calorie restriction
- Activates sirtuins
- Powerful antioxidant
- Anti-aging
- Anti-cancer
- Supports brain function
- Supports heart health
- Longevity vitamin
- Improves insulin sensitivity
- Supports healthy cellular function
- Dose: transform, 250 mg daily
- Food sources: grapes, berry fruits, red wine, plums, peanuts

Curcumin

- Powerful anti-inflammatory effects
- Powerful antioxidant effects
- Free-radical scavenger
- Improves arthritis
- Improves heartburn, gas, bloating, gallbladder, liver and kidney, and gut health
- Improves depression
- Improves Alzheimer's
- Decreases the accumulation of beta-amyloid proteins that cause
- Alzheimer's or dementia

- Supports detoxification of heavy metals
- Protects against xenoestrogens (which often cause cancer)
- Protects mitochondria
- Supports cancer apoptosis
- Anti-carcinogenic
- Take with piperine (extract from black pepper) to improve curcumin absorption
- Dose: 400 g daily
- Food source: turmeric

ALA (Alpha-Lipoic Acid)

- Potent free-radical scavenger
- Powerful antioxidant
- Maintains metabolic health
- Builds glutathione
- Crosses the blood—brain barrier to protect brain
- Improves insulin sensitivity, great for type 2 diabetes
- Stimulates glucose uptake, deceases blood sugar levels
- Regenerates other antioxidants, such as vitamins C, E, glutathione, CoQ10
- Supports cardiac health
- Supports healthy mitochondrial function
- Protects against neurotoxicity
- Prevents diabetic neuropathy
- Weak-heavy-metal detoxifier
- Dose: 600 mg daily
- Food sources: spinach, broccoli, liver, red meat, yams, Brussels sprouts, peas

NAD+

- Neuro-protective (helps prevent Alzheimer's disease)
- Cardio-protective
- Restores and supports mitochondria
- Helps improve metabolism
- Increases insulin sensitivity
- Increases energy production
- Repairs DNA
- Maintains and protects healthy DNA
- Activates sirtuins
- Restores brain plasticity
- Daily dose: 250 mg daily

NAC

- Potent antioxidant
- Anti-inflammatory
- Modulates DNA damage
- Builds glutathione
- Powerful detoxifying agent
- Daily dose: 1.2 mg/day

Probiotics

- Maintains good bacteria balance in the gut flora
- Supports natural immune function
- Supports bowel regularity
- Supports balance of healthy flora during and post antibiotic therapy
- Reduces candida albicans
- Dose: 30 billion CFU daily
- Food sources: olives, sauerkraut, kimchi, tempeh, miso, sourdough bread, yogurts and dark chocolate.

K2

- Promotes healthy blood clotting
- Bone-building
- Reduces arterial stiffening
- Prevents and reduces heart disease, heart attacks and strokes
- Prevents osteoporosis
- Increases insulin sensitivity
- Best to take form of MK-7 with vitamin D3
- Dose: 90 mcg
- Food sources: fermented vegetables such as sauerkraut, organic soybeans, soft and hard cheeses

Vitamin D3

- Powerful anti-inflammatory properties
- Prevents fracture risk
- A pro-hormone, not a vitamin, so a powerful systemic hormone effect
- Helps body defend against any infection
- Improves muscle weakness
- Improves fat cell metabolism, reducing risk of obesity
- Improves insulin sensitivity, reducing type 2 diabetes
- Enhances defense against cancer
- Enhances autophagy
- Reduces autoimmune response
- Low levels associated with depression, anxiety, Alzheimer's and Parkinson's
- Protects brain neuronal decay
- Dose: 4,000 IU daily
- Source: Sun exposure, cod liver oil, cold-water fatty fish, eggs, mushrooms, clarified butter (ghee)

Omega-3 Fatty Acids

- Supports cardiac health, prevents strokes and heart attacks, lowers blood pressure
- Improves and protects against diabetes
- Improves joint pain
- Improves mood disorder (depression and anxiety)
- Supports healthy glucose metabolism and fights insulin resistance
- Neuro-protective, especially DHA fats
- Anti-inflammatory
- Protects against bone loss
- Dose: 1,000–2,000 mg daily
- Food sources: flaxseed oil, virgin olive oil, cod liver oil, anchovy oil, cold-water fish, such as salmon, tuna, sardines, sturgeon

Magnesium

- Essential for over 300 enzymatic reactions
- Necessary for energy production
- Maintains heart health
- Maintains bones
- Maintains teeth
- Metabolizes carbs, fats, proteins and sugar
- Supports healthy muscle function
- Supports healthy nerve function
- Supports healthy bowel function
- Natural calming agent
- Dose: 400 mg
- Food sources: green leafy vegetables, soaked Brazilian nuts, almonds, quinoa, organic soybeans

CoQ10

- Generates cellular energy
- Supports cardiac health
- Supports brain health
- Supports healthy immune response
- Quenches free radicals
- Dose: 200 mg daily

DIM (Diindolylmethane)

- Promotes healthy estrogen metabolism, shifts the metabolism pathway to produce 2-hydroxyestrone, a safe estrogen
- Protects against xenoestrogens (which often cause cancer)
- Powerful detoxifying agent that neutralizes the damaging effects of estrogen
- Promotes beneficial estrogen metabolism in women, preventing and protecting against breast, uterine, endometrial, ovarian and cervical cancers
- Protects against breast cancer in men and lowers excess estrogens in men
- Dose: 250 mg daily
- Diet source: cruciferous vegetables

S-Acytle Glutathione

- Potent antioxidant
- Protects body from oxidative stress
- Maintains cellular functions
- Restores and supports mitochondrial health
- Supports healthy immune response
- Detoxifying agent
- Enhances vitamins C and E antioxidant activity
- Dose: 200 mg
- Diet source: asparagus, onions, broccoli, apples, bananas, oranges

B Complex

- Helps maintain memory
- Decreases homocysteine
- Detoxifies estrogen

Vitamin B12

- Mood-enhancing
- Memory-enhancing
- Energy production
- Dose: 3,000 ug daily
- Diet source: lean organic meats, wild fish, clams, mussels, eggs

Soluble Fiber

- Reduces bad cholesterol
- Promotes healthy gut bacteria and flora
- Decreases insulin resistance and improves type 2 diabetes
- Decreases risk of colon cancer
- Dose: females 21–25 grams daily; males 30–38 grams daily
- Diet sources: berries, bananas, citrus fruit, apples, pears, plums, all veggies, mushrooms, nuts and seeds, oatmeal, buckwheat, quinoa, whole grain rice, barley, lentils, chickpeas, beans, peas, popcorn

Zinc

- Strong antioxidant
- Potent immune stimulant
- Essential for over 200 enzymatic reactions
- Critical for preventing benign prostate hypertrophy and prostate cancer in men; lowers excessive estrogens in men
- Involved in sperm production and prevents impotency

- Important for hair and skin
- Reduces acne
- Dose: 25 mg daily
- Food sources: abundant in most nuts and seeds, grains, beans, egg yolk, chicken, free-range beef, oysters

Quercetin

- Powerful anti-inflammatory effects
- Powerful antioxidant effects
- Sirtuin activator
- Free-radical scavenger
- Enhances insulin production to help prevent type 2 diabetes
- Dose: 250 mg daily
- Food sources: apples, berries, broccoli, onions, grapes, tea, kale

Vitamin C

- Water soluble
- We don't make it!
- Promotes collagen formation
- Energy production
- Protects against free radicals and prevents cancer
- Potent antioxidant that protects DNA from free radicals and mutations
- Prevents allergies
- White blood cells need it to defend the body against bacteria and viruses
- Helps balance adrenal glands and reduce stress
- Dose: 1,000–2,000 mg daily, get buffered vitamin C to not upset stomach
- Food sources: berries, citrus, green leafy greens, avocados, cruciferous vegetables

L-Theonine

- Natural sleeping aid
- Decreases stress and anxiety
- Great calming effect, short acting
- Dose: 200–600 mg every 4 to 6 hours
- Food sources: green tea

Melatonin

- A hormone the body makes to regulate our circadian rhythm
- Potent antioxidant that prevents cancer
- Natural sleeping aid
- Immunity builder
- Helps with production of growth hormone
- Decreases cortisol
- Dose: take between 1–3 mg at bedtime

Astragalus Root/ Ashwagandha Root

- Activates telomerase to preserve telomeres
- Improves memory
- Improves alertness
- Decreases stress
- Helps damaged neurons of brain regenerate (shown in lab studies)
- Dose: 250 mg daily

Phosphatidylserine

- Increases neurotransmitters in the brain to improve mood, depression, anxiety
- Helps maintain memory and cognitive function
- Improves attention and concentration

- Improves ability to cope with stress
- Decreases cortisol
- Dose: 300 mg at bedtime
- Food sources: fish, rice, organic soy and dark leafy greens

WHAT ARE SYSTEMIC ENZYMES?

We are born with over 3,000 enzymes. By the time we are 27 years old, we've used up most of our supply, and innate production diminishes. The body has over 7,000 vital enzymatic reactions that do just about everything: growth, reproduction, digestion, immunity and metabolism. Chemical reactions in the body are generally a slow process, and enzymes "speed up" the chemical reactions in the body. Enzymes control and eliminate inflammation, regulate metabolism and promote natural healing. Healing is crippled without enzymes.

In Asia and Europe, systemic enzymes are heavily used to maintain healthy body aging, healing and cancer prevention. Enzymes are naturally anti-inflammatory. They break down the food we eat and gets it ready for digestion and absorption. Enzymes are naturally occurring in the foods we eat, especially organic raw vegetables. Processing and overheating kills enzymes found in whole foods. Studies show that systemic enzymes can help decrease inflammation and scar tissue. Taking systemic enzymes reduces inflammation, reduces the formation of excessive scar tissue, aids in blood cleansing, boosts immune function and helps fight viruses.

Cancer cells stick to cell walls and multiply while hiding, trying to escape being recognized by the body's innate immune system. Cancer does so by coating itself with adhesive fibrin, about 15 layers thicker than a healthy normal cell. This helps cancer cells grow unrecognized as the "enemy." Researchers Freund and Kaminer suggest that cancer can grow in the absence of enzymes and that enzymes can serve as "blocking factors" for cancers. Enzymes have proteolytic properties to strip cancer of its fibrin, so that the cancer is more vulnerable to anti-cancer treatments.

WHAT IS VITAMIN D3?

Vitamin D3 is one of the most important vitamins to take daily. Vitamin D functions more as a hormone, rather than a vitamin. It is made from cholesterol, just like other hormones in the body and functions as a prohormone.

The sun is the main source of vitamin D. Our skin absorbs sun and our body manufactures vitamin D3. As we age, it's harder to make and levels decline. Wearing sunscreen blocks vitamin D formation. Food is not a significant source of vitamin D either. Vitamin D3 is also the powerful, active and beneficial form of vitamin D. Supplementation is best.

As a preventative, anti-aging physician, I recommend optimal levels, not just normal levels, of vitamin D3. The optimal level is 50–80 nmol/L. It is most critical to have your doctor check your vitamin D3 levels and make sure it's in a healthy range. Most people have never had their vitamin D3 levels checked. And, most people are quite deficient in vitamin D3, a totally preventable epidemic.

Sunlight is a healthy way to also get your daily dose. Just 15 to 30 minutes a day in high sun provides a daily dose of vitamin D. This actually is equivalent to 10,000 to 15,000 IU of vitamin D3. Sadly, the recommended reference dosing is only 600 IU per day. Most experts would recommend closer to 4,000–6,000 IU per day. Please have your vitamin D3 levels monitored by your physician because, as with any of the other hormones, monitoring for balance and safety is important. Patients with chronic conditions may need more and should be monitored by checking blood levels.

Researchers have now discovered vitamin D receptors throughout all our body tissues: brain, gut, breasts, prostate, bone, colon, muscle, pancreas, lungs and white blood cells. Vitamin D provides cellular function, growth and gene expression, targeting over 2,000 genes in our cells.

Most people think of bones when they think of vitamin D. Vitamin D is critical for bone health too, and vitamin D3 prevents bone fractures and maintains bone density. It also helps calcium absorption in the small intestine and helps put the calcium into the bones. However, even more incredible, vitamin D3 is a powerful immune-stimulant. It boosts our immune system to have anticancer activation at all times. It is also powerful in preventing insulin resistance and type 2 diabetes. The pancreas has vitamin D receptors that help with insulin secretion. It also helps lower blood pressure.

Over 2,500 published studies confirm that higher vitamin D3 levels have profound benefits, preventing cancer formation, especially breast, colon and prostate. According to Dr. Michael Hollick, the leading authority on vitamin D, optimal dosing of D3 can reduce risks of heart attacks by as much as 50%, decrease breast, colon and prostate cancers by about the same percent, and reduce the common flu and cold as much as 90%! Dr. Hollick's book, *The Vitamin D Solution*, is a great resource for learning about the powerful effects of vitamin D3 on the body. He explains how limited sun exposure and wearing sun protection is one of the major causes of a pandemic vitamin D deficiency. Based on research that vitamin D reduces heart disease, cancer and diabetes, Dr. Hollick believes, *"We could probably decrease health-care costs across the board by 25% if everyone had optimal vitamin D status."*

In the *Journal of the National Cancer Institute*, a collaborative, international study of over 20 medical centers have found that higher circulating vitamin D3 levels correlate with significantly lower risks of colorectal cancer. Colon cancer is the third most common cancer in the U.S. and third leading cause of cancer deaths.

A study in 2011 from Germany reported that lower levels of vitamin D3 levels were inversely related to breast cancer recurrence and increased mortality. Increased vitamin D3 levels were cancer-protective. Scientists postulate that vitamin D3 may lower cancer risk by regulating cell growth.

Research shows vitamin D3 improves serotonin levels, improving depression and even chronic fatigue. Optimizing vitamin D3 increases energy and helps you to cope with stress. Most impressive, a study of 498 women over a seven-year span showed those with the highest intake of vitamin D had a 77% reduced risk of getting Alzheimer's disease.

Vitamin D3 also diminishes the risks of Parkinson's disease, multiple sclerosis, and other dementias. It preserves bone health, prevents inflammation, osteoporosis, both type 1 and type 2 diabetes, depression, heart disease, hypertension, back pain, muscle pain and autoimmune disease.

Vitamin D3 has extraordinary preventive powers we all need!

CHAPTER 19

Sex, Orgasms & Healthy Relationships— Preserve Youth and Longevity

Self-love is the source of all other loves.
—Pierre Corneille

RELATIONSHIPS AFFECT OUR HEALTH. RESEARCH SHOWS THAT married people tend to live longer. An amazing TED Talk by Robert Waldinger called *"What Makes a Good Life? Lessons from the Longest Study on Happiness"* is an absolute must-listen. It is 13 minutes of valuable insights from a 75-year study that reveals that happiness and long life come from fulfilling relationships, not fame and money.

Loneliness, the New Epidemic

We can live without religion and meditation,
but we cannot survive without human affection.

—Dalai Lama

Loneliness is a health risk. Studies show that lonely people tend to have increased cortisol levels, the "stress hormone" that's responsible for high inflammation, impaired immune function, frequent sickness, poor sleep, high blood pressure, heart disease and premature death. A study from BYU (Brigham Young University) found that social isolation or chronic loneliness actually has as big an impact on mortality risk factors similar to smoking and is twice as dangerous as obesity. A newer study of 20,000 U.S. adults, 18 years and older, has disturbing new findings:

- One in six adults have some form of mental health condition, causing them to miss work.
- Generation Z (ages 18 to 22) and Millennials (ages 23 to 27) are the loneliest, worse than all other age groups, and report to be in the worst health.
- Students are lonelier than retirees.
- Almost half of Americans reported feeling lonesome, regardless of gender or race.
- Loneliness is reported to have the same impact as smoking 15 cigarettes per day and is regarded more dangerous to health than obesity.

The "I" in illness is isolation, and the
crucial letters in wellness are "we."

—Unknown

Loneliness has become an epidemic. In fact, as of January 2018, the United Kingdom announced the creation of a Minister for Loneliness role within its government. The commission was created after a report last year was released declaring that 15–20% of British adults were "often or always feeling lonely." Their task is to involve these lonely people and have them engaged in community gatherings and events.

Brigham Young University psychology and neuroscience professor Julianne Holt-Lunstad says, "*Loneliness epidemic is developing in the United States, too—and the U.S. should consider following Britain's lead in making loneliness a public-health priority."* I agree; we need to identify and help teens and young adults, especially, with overcoming these feelings of disconnect.

In this internet era of social media, informational technologies have dominated our culture and how we communicate. Due to internet dating, selfies, texting, emailing, and HD (high definition) video games, people have lost the skill of social grace and manners. People isolate themselves and communicate over phone, text, and Twitter all too frequently. Poor communication skills, poor eye contact, difficulty connecting emotionally or verbally to another human being has become a challenge for many. We are brought closer together with technology, from all over the world but, ironically, have a greater sense of loneliness.

Technology isn't all to blame. We need to limit technology time and have more people time. We don't interact as much by touch, energy, chemical (as in, with chemistry) or eye connection. We've become more robotic, mechanical. People feel alone, empty, numb and lack empathy. There is too much noise with the internet and, with it off, it is too lonely, boring, uncomfortable.

Disconnect from TV, internet, and social media. Connect to humanity, learn to practice compassion and empathy. Go out of your comfort zone and work out outside, go for a walk, make new friends and connections, and spend time in nature. Volunteer at an animal shelter, nursing home, or hospital. Join a workout group, art class, or any class to be around people with similar interests. Visit the library, a museum, or go to the theater and art shows. Don't watch Youtube videos on "how to"—go to a cooking class with other people, learn painting, piano, or tennis from a person in real time.

It is important to have live, interactive, social connections, to friends, family and community. Strengthen bonds with family and friends. Get a rescue cat or dog—it is a great way to get immediate companionship. Disengage from electronics and re-engage in society. Learn to become comfortable being alone. It is healthy to value time alone without feeling lonely. Be bored, still, quiet, meditate, read, and revel in it. Blaise Pascal wrote, *"All of humanity's problems stem from man's inability to sit quietly in a room alone."*

Benefits of Sex and Orgasms

*"Sex" is as important as eating or drinking and
we ought to allow the one appetite to be satisfied
with as little restraint or false modesty as the other.*

—Marquis de Sade

Benefits of intimacy are lasting happiness and health. According to a 2014 Johns Hopkins University study, couples ages 58 to 85 who had frequent sex or sexual intimacy as little as once a month had greater marital satisfaction and happier relationships than those who hadn't had sex in over a year. Oxytocin, the "love hormone," along with the other endorphins, is released during intimacy, creating healthy bonding and cementing a relationship.

Regular sexual activity gives you more energy and motivation, and prevents depression, improves the immune system, relieves pain, improves relationship bonding, decreases anxiety, lowers blood pressure, strengthens heart tissue, and induces sleep. Data suggests that a regular sex life is two to three times a week. I advise patients once a week is minimum and three times ideal. Frequent sex preserves the brain, sleep, and immune system, extends lifespan and cements a healthy relationship.

Orgasms and regular sex also make you look younger too. At a 2013 British Psychological Society annual meeting, researchers presented a study that found subjects, 40 to 50 years old, who had sex three times a week, looked 4 to 5 years younger than their counterparts who had less.

Orgasms have significant neurological benefits with a surge of endorphins, serotonin and dopamine levels skyrocketing. Dopamine is released from the left brain, serotonin from the right brain. A 2010 study from Princeton University showed that rats with more sexual activity had increased neuronal growth in the hippocampus region of the brain. This is the key learning and memory center of the brain. The brain is activated with improved memory, creativity and motivation, all super-charging the brain.

Orgasms are a great way to reduce stress and anxiety. A 2005 Scottish study showed that subjects who engaged in regular sexual activity over two weeks had lower blood pressure, anxiety and stress levels, as compared to their counterpart subjects who had no sex for two weeks. The sexually active group also had a much better perception of stress.

Orgasms also reduce emotional and physical pain by replacing pain with pleasure and inducing an endorphin surge. Joint and muscle pain, PMS and headaches diminish. Instead of self-medicating with pain meds, sleeping aids or alcohol, engage in a healthy sexual release instead.

Regular sex and orgasms boost the immune system and protect against cancer. Researchers from Wilkes University reported college students who had sex 1 to 2 times a week had 30% higher levels of immunoglobulin (IgA), in their saliva as compared to students who had infrequent sex. IgA is an antibody that plays a crucial role in the immune function of mucous membranes, especially in the respiratory and digestive tracts. IgA protects us from viruses, such as the flu, and microbes that infect the gut health. Some research suggests that men who have more frequent ejaculations have a decreased risk of prostate cancer. A French study reported that women who had sex at least once a month had a decreased risk of developing breast cancer.

Orgasms produce longevity. There are scientific data supporting a busier sex life means a longer life. One notable study concluded that having 100 orgasms per year can increase life expectancy by 3 to 8 years. And having two orgasms per week decreased a person's death rate by 68%, significantly lower than their counterparts that had orgasms once a month. A 10-year Welsh study following 900 men, ages 45 to 59, reported that men with a high frequency of orgasms had a 50% reduction in mortality rate. The more orgasms, the lower the mortality, and the fewer the orgasms, the higher mortality.

In a 25-year study conducted by Duke University, researchers found the frequency of sex was inverse to mortality in men (more sex, less death). In women, the enjoyment of intercourse was found to be inversely related to mortality (more sexually-related pleasure, less death). It seems, based on studies, quantity matters to men, and quality is more paramount for women. Researchers reported that in a case-controlled study following middle-aged women, it showed women who were dissatisfied with the quality of sex, primarily due to premature ejaculation or impotence of their partners, were at an increased risk of acute myocardial infarction.

Orgasms are also a natural sleep aid. I tell patients that an orgasm is the best way to start your sleep. Prolactin, a relaxation hormone, along with the other endorphins induces a more restful sleep. A study in 2000 showed that 32% of females who masturbated fell asleep much better than their non-masturbating counterparts. Orgasms are a great healthy bonding experience with your partner. They recharge the brain with "happy joy joy" feelings, increase your innate immune system and give you great sleep.

The only thing about masturbation
to be ashamed of is doing it badly.
—Sigmund Freud

Surveys have shown people of all ages, in or out of relationships, masturbate regularly. Interestingly, a study in *Playboy* found that 72% of married men masturbate and a study in *Redbook* found that 68% of their married female readers masturbate. Self-pleasure should not be a behavior of shame, especially in single people; it's the safest sex. Masturbation prevents a single person from rushing into an unhealthy relationship for the wrong reasons, and they can still get the health benefits of orgasms.

CHAPTER 20

Optimum Mental Health

There is no illness of the body apart from the mind.
—Socrates

NEGATIVE THINKING DESTROYS THE BODY AND SPIRIT. Pessimism leads to a poor immune system and depression. Depression is obsessing or being stuck in the past. Anxiety is consistently worrying about the future. It all leads to overthinking, less doing, a poorer immune system, disease formation, and a shorter life.

Clinical depression and anxiety are serious medical problems that are critical to evaluate, especially if hormone-related. When men and women start declining in testosterone and estrogen levels, they become more vulnerable to depression and anxiety. If someone had a history of mood disorders and were stable on medical treatment and suddenly feel worse with menopause or andropause, that's because these conditions become worse with decreasing hormones. Such a person becomes more vulnerable to stressors, feeling higher, uncontrolled levels of depression, anxiety and worsening insomnia.

Nearly one in four women in their 40s and 50s have been pre-scribed antidepressants. If you've never had a history of being treated for clinical depression, anxiety or insomnia, and it all starts after age 35 to 40, it's more likely symptoms of your declining hormones. This needs to be evaluated thoroughly before starting on antidepressants or anti-anxiety medications and, especially, addictive sleeping aids.

Conventionally, most women or men going through menopause or andropause immediately are given such medications to cope, to Band-Aid their symptoms, rather than to truly treat and resolve their symptoms. Lack of estrogen in women, and testosterone in men, leads to depression, anxiety, panic attacks, insomnia and feelings of irritability, frustration, lack of focus, and proneness to negativity and pessimism.

It is so important to evaluate each patient, listen to them, learn their medical history, check their hormone panel, and restore and bal-ance their hormones instead of quickly prescribing new lifetime drugs and diagnoses. Restoring hormones, in my experience, helps people need less or no anti-depressants, especially if they've never been on them prior to menopause or andropause. Not only does it give back mental calm, but also sleep, energy, and sex drive; it also empowers them with motivation for weight loss.

It is critical for your well-being to get help for depression, whether it is linked to your menopause/andropause, or not, but especially if it is linked to declining hormones and aging. Studies have reported that depression is linked to high blood pressure, cardiac arrhythmias, high cortisol levels, Alzheimer's disease and heart attacks. Extreme pessimism is also associated with later onset of dementia and heart disease. Studies also show that people with both type 2 diabetes and depression have a higher mortality rate than having just one of the disorders. Depressed people tend to be pessimists.

A Finnish study followed cynics and pessimists for eight years and found them to be at a higher risk for dementia. Cynics, those that generally see the worst in others, were more likely to develop demen-tia compared to their more trusting peers.

BECOME AN ETERNAL OPTIMIST!

Some people grumble that roses have thorns.
I am grateful that thorns have roses.

—Alphonse Karr

Recent studies have shown that optimists, or positive thinkers, tend to be healthier and live longer lives. Researchers at the University of Illinois found that positive people have better blood sugar levels, cholesterol levels, and body mass indexes than their pessimistic counterparts. They were also more active and didn't smoke. They concluded that optimists had less heart disease. Numerous studies have shown optimism protects heart heath and lowers blood pressure. Another study from University of Pittsburgh also found that optimists are less likely to die from a variety of diseases, including heart disease, cancer, depression and diabetes.

In another study, researchers found that optimists had a better immune system, and the stronger their optimism, the stronger their immunity. When they exposed volunteer subjects to a common respiratory virus, the positive personality peers were less likely to develop viral infections, as opposed their negative-thinking peers.

A series of studies have found a link between optimism and longevity. One study followed college students for 40 years and found that the optimists were less likely to die; even the optimists that had cancer and heart attacks survived longer. Optimism helps people cope with disease better and recover from surgery. The researchers suggested that those who expected better outcomes coped with stress better, and this had a positive effect on their overall health and longevity.

Optimism has been linked to living well and living longer. In a 2012 study of 243 centenarians, researchers found that most of them looked at life "through rose-colored glasses." Optimists survive disease and cancer with better outcomes, have better pain tolerance and live longer, regardless of income level or overall health implications.

Having a positive attitude and finding the "silver lining," no matter what might be ailing you, can boost your mental and physical health.

A man is but the product of his thoughts —
what he thinks, he becomes.

—Gandhi

What's exciting is that there is a psychological phenomenon called "emotional contagion," which is a theory that people catch feelings from one another, just like they would catch a cold from one another. Basically, our emotions rub off onto one another. If you're optimistic and happy, you infect others with it; if you're cynical and pessimistic, you also spread that. These are non-verbal cues; they don't need to be verbal. It's the expressions you carry on your face and show in your eyes. You can transfer your emotions to others and, likewise, they can transfer theirs to you as well.

Be highly selective and detox the negative people and their effects on your mental and physical health. Think about your emotions and become aware of how you transfer them to the people you love, live with and work with in your life. It is important you spread optimism, joy and smiles; these are healthy vibes. You are responsible for what you think, feel and do. What you put out there comes back to you!

ACCOUNTABILITY

If you do not love yourself entirely and
actively ensure your own needs are met,
you will find it difficult to do the same for others.

—Zaid Dahhaj

This is critical to understand: we are self-capable and reliant to take care of ourselves and to not search for someone else to take care of our needs. We must look for happiness within ourselves. Others are usually unreliable, and it is not their responsibility to fulfill us. Our partners and loved ones can add to our happiness, but they cannot be the main source. We must find ways to be purposeful, to give back and contribute to ourselves, every day. Being proactive and intentional in taking care of our health, proper eating, exercising, emotional outlets and diffusion of stress all invites happiness within ourselves.

PRACTICE MINDFULNESS

Do not anticipate trouble or worry about what
may never happen. Keep in the sunlight.

—Benjamin Franklin

Depression is obsessing or being stuck in the past. Anxiety is worrying about the future. Practice being in the present. Practice mindfulness, a state of being in what is, as it is.

How do we start practicing mindfulness? First, recognize that we all have habits. Some are mindless repetitions, some are good, and some are bad habits. Start becoming aware of your thoughts, habits and reactions, not just mindlessly responding. We are wired to hold onto negative moments or thoughts, so become aware of these negative thoughts, how you talk to yourself, your fears. Slow down, breathe, and convert negative to positive thoughts. Start adopting responsibility to change and commit to being better. Monitor your thought patterns and habitual cyclical patterns.

Take a meditation class. Meditation helps clear the mind and reintroduce calm, decluttering it and staying in the present. Mindful meditation helps restore calm. Start breaking negative thinking—catch yourself in the thought and put a positive thought in its place. Your brain is soil for your body, so cultivating positive thoughts cultivates healthy and positive effects.

Be present, savor the present. Feel what you feel now, focus entirely on the present. Enjoy positive moments, like watching the sunset, drinking a great cup of coffee, watching your kids play, walking your dog, watching the basketball playoffs... Engage all the senses you've been gifted with—smelling, tasting, touching, seeing, hearing.

Have gratitude for what you do have in your life. Savor it fully. Do it every day. Appreciate positive events, no matter how small they are, daily. Practicing daily enjoyment of positive moments and repeating daily empowers positivity to be a new habit, forming new positive memories. Even with difficult days, find a positive event or moment.

To truly feel good, be good. That means making efforts to be better by action: to eat better, exercise, meditate and to commit to healthier, mindful habits.

CHAPTER 21

Distress Is an Age-Accelerator

It is not the strongest of the species which survives,
or the most intelligent which survives. It is the one
which is the most adaptable to change.

—Charles Darwin

STRESS IS THE EFFECT WE FEEL WHEN WE'RE FACED WITH challenges, and we've all had them. Most people are unaware, however, that there are two forms of stress, eustress and distress. We cannot control stressors; we can only control our perception of stress.

Following are some descriptions of each type of stressor.

EUSTRESS

- Good stress
- Increases endorphins
- Increases immune system
- Increases energy and motivation, excitement
- Increases creativity in the brain and thinking

- Preserves the alkaline body
- Short-term
- Feels exhilarating/energizing
- Increases performance
- Examples: promotion at work, new move, new baby, new projects, party, vacation or event planning, starting a new business, retiring, training for an event, a wedding

DISTRESS

- Bad stress
- Decreases endorphins
- Lowers the immune system
- Depletes energy and causes fatigue
- Increases anxiety and depressive feelings
- Lowers pH of body, lowers oxygen in body, shallow breathing
- Short-term or long-term
- Decreases performance, emotional depletion
- Feels unpleasant/painful
- Can lead to mental and physical problems, emotional depletion
- Examples: death of a loved one, divorce, deadlines at work, arguments with loved ones or in relationships, being late, health challenges, getting sick or injured, financial hardships, poor sleeping, low job satisfaction

Stress is inevitable. The perception of stress is important to how the body responds. The body supports the brain's perception of stress.

> *If you are irritated by every rub,*
> *how will you be polished?*
> —Rumi

Distress is an age-accelerator. It is focusing on fear of the unknown and lack of faith that life has something good to offer you. This mental conditioning is recycled again and again, leading to a feeling of doom. As previously discussed, this chronic distress releases the bad hormone cortisol. As cortisol levels increase and persist, your body produces more free radicals, handicapping your immune system and leading to premature aging, decaying and diseases.

Chronic stress causes weight gain with a stubborn fat that won't burn with proper exercise and eating. It interrupts deep sleeping and disrupts brain function, as well as thyroid and hormonal release and balance throughout the body. Abundant research supports that chronic distress increases heart attack rates, strokes and cancer risk. About 75–90% of visits to the primary care doctor are related to the effects of distress.

We will be exposed to stress, ongoing. The solution isn't to eliminate stress; rather, it is to change our perception of it. We need to respond by "releasing" stress, not keeping it locked in and causing internal bodily damage.

Accepting responsibility for how you respond to stressors is critical to changing your behavior patterns. Trying to see the silver lining in the worst situations and retain a desire to overcome an obstacle helps your body diffuse the negative consequences of distress. Become mindful of how you interpret stress, and see it as a challenge, not a punishment.

Start slowly and be consistent. Using stress constructively to cultivate growth takes practice and mindfulness. This helps foster a healthy body and brain, not one full of sickness and disease. Start with proper breathing.

Proper breathing is a great skill to learn. When we get nervous, upset or stressed, we tend to shallow breathe. Learning to breathe out stress helps us to cope better and releases the negative energy and tension, instead of torturing our body and brain with it.

BREATHING

It's not stress that kills us. It is our reaction to it.

—Hans Selye

We may not be able to control the stressors; however, we can absolutely control how we respond to stress. Most people do not realize that they are in full control of their breathing. Many don't ever think about breathing because the body just automatically does it. When we get anxious, we short breathe; this causes more anxiety because shallow breaths cause lactic acid buildup, cortisol production, and digestive problems. Deep breathing and oxygen restore calm, release anxiety, increase alertness and energy, alkalize the blood and ease muscle tension, heart palpitations and gastrointestinal distress.

My favorite breathing relaxing technique that I recommend to my patients was developed by Dr. Andrew Weil, an alternative medicine guru. His technique is called "4-7-8 Relaxing Breath Exercise." It's easy, and you could do it anywhere. He describes it as a natural tranquilizer for the nervous system. I couldn't agree more.

Dr. Weil's 4-7-8 Breathing Method

- Sit up or lie down with your back straight. Place the tip of your tongue against the ridge of tissue just behind your upper front teeth. Keep your tongue positioned there the entire time.
- Exhale completely through your mouth, making a whoosh sound.
- With your mouth closed, inhale quietly through your nose to a mental count of four.
- Hold your breath for a count of seven.

- Exhale completely through your mouth, making a whoosh sound to a count of eight.
- This is one breath. Repeat three more times. Do this anytime you feel upset, stressed out or just to pass time. Repeat as needed.

LAUGHTER

Humor is the balancing stick
that allows us to walk the tightrope of life.
—John F. Kennedy

Laughter has been known as the "best medicine." It sure is. There's nothing like a great deep belly laugh! It is a great way to celebrate life and cope with the bad. People who laugh more live longer and tend to be more optimistic. They find reasons to laugh even when it's not that funny, and they like to make people happy.

Females tend to laugh more than males—126% more! Men tend to be more laugh-getters. A study in *Psychology Today* reported, "*The laughter of the female is the critical index of a healthy relationship.*" Women need to keep laughing to preserve a happy family because their laughs are more contagious and have a powerful effect.

Laughing also boosts the immune system. Laughter activates T-cells, natural immune cells that fight off sickness. Those who laugh more get fewer colds and get sick less often. The endorphins released from laughing are the body's natural painkillers. The endorphins are a "natural high" that also help lower cortisol levels and help to cope and reduce tension, stress and depression. Laughter diffuses anger and anxiety. Actually, it makes you feel good all over. Research shows that laughter in relationships declines dramatically as people age. So, it is important to keep each other amused. There was a study published in a geriatric journal that found that laughter therapy reduced depression in the elderly and improved their sense of well-being.

Laughing has similar benefits to deep breathing; you use your diaphragm, abs, heart and lungs in both. You also have to release all the air in your lungs and take in oxygen-rich air doing both. According to the Mayo Clinic, laughter is heart-healthy and lowers your blood pressure too. People love to be around laughter—it is good energy and makes people happy and smile.

CHAPTER 22

Prayer Is Powerful!

*In whatever you do today, remember GOD is beside you. And no
matter what comes your way, remember, HIS hand will guide you.*

—Unknown

IS YOUR FEAR GREATER THAN YOUR FAITH? FAITH AND PRAYER
are the most popular form of alternative medicine. It's about having
hope, to dwell outside of yourself, to surrender.

BENEFITS OF PRAYER

Regardless of religious preference, having a higher spirit to believe
in helps people cope with pain, stress, cancer and disease. Research
supports that prayer improves health and lengthens life. Dartmouth
Medical School researchers found that patients with regular prayer
habits who underwent elective heart surgery were three times more
likely to recover than those that didn't. And patients who prayed regularly before heart surgery experienced less depression and anxiety
afterwards, according to studies from University of Washington
Health Sciences and the University of Pittsburgh. Patients that prayed

only after surgery did not have the same benefits in either study as those who prayed before and after surgery.

A study in *The Journals of Gerontology* reported data following 4,000 senior citizens. It found that those who prayed or meditated coped better with illness and lived longer than their counterparts. Another study funded by the National Institutes of Health (NIH) found that people who prayed daily had a 40% reduction in blood pressure compared to those who didn't have regular prayer practices.

Numerous studies have shown how regular prayer decreases chronic pain, improves mood and recovery after major surgeries, lowers blood pressure, improves stress coping, and improves the immune system. Prayer is positive and powerful.

CHAPTER 23

Stress Diffusion

*It is how people respond to stress that determines
whether they will profit from misfortune or be miserable.*

—Mihaly Csikszentmihalyi

I RECOMMEND TO MY PATIENTS THE FOLLOWING TOOLS TO
diffuse stress. Stress is part of life, so we must learn to see its value
and release the energy back out. Convert the bad energy into good
energy and surrender to faith and optimism. Make sure your hormones are also balanced and try the following activities to diffuse
your stress. You can choose the ones you like or do them all. Perhaps,
you may already do some of them, so do more. Keep doing as many
as you can, as often as you can. Turn pain into pleasure. Here are the
practices I recommend.

1. Laughter
2. Deep breathing exercises
3. Taking regular vacations or taking a day off

4. Smiling—it's contagious
5. Limit blue light from computers, phones, and video games first thing in the mornings and after 6PM. Try to disconnect from technology more and engage with family and friends more often.
6. Grounding: walking barefoot on grass or sand
7. Adopt the victor role, not the victim role
8. Prayer
9. Mindful meditation
10. Yoga
11. Regular exercise
12. Massage treatments
13. Reading
14. Sex, intimacy and orgasms
15. Sleep 7 to 8 hours
16. Hobbies—relaxing and having fun; cooking, fishing, gardening, drawing, singing, dancing, volunteering
17. Journaling—gratitude journal
18. Therapy
19. Essential oils
20. Acupuncture
21. Social support and engagement
23. Listening to music
24. Going for a walk
25. Cultivate positive thinking. Look for the silver lining.
26. Practice mindfulness, being in the present moment.
27. Drink chamomile tea; it helps to calm nerves.

These supplements are also excellent to help with stress management. Take them regularly, and after 6 to 8 weeks, you'll likely appreciate positive results.

1. Holy basil—1,200 mg daily
2. L-theonine—200 mg, repeat every 4 to 6 hours as needed
3. Phosphatidylserine—300 mg daily
4. Ashwagandha—250 mg daily

A vigorous five-mile walk will do more good
for an unhappy but otherwise healthy adult
than all the medicine and psychology in the world.

— Paul Dudley White, M.D.,
prominent American cardiologist

CHAPTER 24

Optimizing Cancer Prevention

Treatment without prevention
is simply unsustainable.
—Bill Gates

CANCER IS THE SECOND LEADING CAUSE OF DEATH IN Americans, second only to heart disease. Cancer continues to be a worldwide killer, regardless of the enormous amount of cancer research development. According to the National Cancer Institute, an estimated 38.4% of Americans will be diagnosed with cancer at some point in their lifetime. That means about one in three people will be diagnosed with cancer.

The National Institute of Health (NIH) further reported the overall cancer death rates in the U.S. have declined by 25% since 1990. As the overall cancer death rate has declined, the number of cancers has increased, and few cancers have been stabilized and have even increased. In 2018, they estimate 1,735,350 new cases of cancer will be diagnosed in the U.S. The most common cancers diagnosed will be breast, lung, prostate, colon and melanoma skin cancer.

GENETICS VS. LIFESTYLE

According to the National Cancer Institute, only 5–10% of all cancer cases are caused by hereditary or genetic defects. An astounding 90–95% of cancer cases are rooted in environment and lifestyle choices! Lifestyle factors include cigarette smoking, a diet based on meat, animal fats and processed foods, excessive alcohol consumption, stress, obesity, and lack of exercise. Environment factors include excessive sun exposure, food additives, dioxins, pesticides, radiation exposure, nitrates, and toxins in cosmetics, plastics and air pollution. Evidence shows that of all the cancer-related deaths, 25–30% are due to tobacco, 30–40% due to diet and obesity, and 15–20% due to infectious agents, usually viral.

I believe that we must apply our current science to vigorously focus on cancer prevention and cancer recurrence education. We have to be accountable for our part in cancer and disease formation. Following, I have detailed powerful methods for cancer prevention, recurrence and existing cancer intervention.

CHAPTER 25

Increasing Cancer Immunity

*Too many of us are not living our dreams
because we are living our fears.*

—Les Brown

THE FOLLOWING ARE NECESSARY STEPS YOU CAN TAKE TO intentionally increase your innate cancer immunity.

FIX GUT HEALTH!

Death begins in the colon.

—Eli Metchnifoff, PhD,
Nobel Prize winner

Gut health is everything. The chapter dedicated to gut health is important to review again, as the health of your gut is the basis of disease formation, which leads to your body not being able to ward off cancer.

EAT MORE VEGETABLES AND BE AT AN OPTIMAL WEIGHT!

The doctor of the future will give no medication
but will interest his patients in the care of the human frame,
diet and in the cause and prevention of disease.

—Thomas Edison

The CDC has reported that 40% of cancers are obesity- and diet-related. Obesity is a risk factor for cancer because obesity increases inflammation, raises insulin levels and raises abnormal sex hormones in the blood. These abnormal sex hormones are released from fat cells and can cause cancer cells to grow unchecked. Studies show that two-thirds of people with obesity-related cancer are between 50 to 74 years old when diagnosed, and rates were higher in women. Be accountable. Body fat matters. Healthy total body fat for women is 16–25% and 8–18% for men. Lose weight with regular exercise and eating abundant organic, whole, nutrient-dense foods, especially vegetables and fruits.

By eating vegetables, fruits, whole grains and nuts, you get a large amount of fiber intake. Fiber is a vital nutrient that slows down sugar absorption, lowers cholesterol, decreases food cravings and is heart and cancer-protective. People who eat the most high-fiber foods tend to be the healthiest. According to *The Journal of the American Medical Association*, fiber intake from foods is a good marker for disease risk. Nutritious foods are high in fiber and lower disease risk. Meat, dairy, and foods made from refined sugars and flour (have had their fiber removed) generally do not contain fiber and have a higher disease-risk. Eating leafy, green, nutrient- and fiber-rich vegetables and whole foods is the best predictor of extreme immunity and longevity.

SUGAR IS TOXIC!

Sugar is the most hazardous foodstuff in the American diet.

—Linus Pauling, PhD, twice Nobel Prize Laureate

Professor Otto Warburg, a two-time Nobel Prize Winner in 1931 and 1944, discovered the difference between healthy cells and cancer cells. He said, *"The prime cause of cancer is the replacement of the respiration of oxygen in normal body cells by fermentation of sugar."* What does this mean? That cancer cannot grow or survive without sugar. Cancer is a sugar feeder. Lead scientist, Demetrakopoulos, whose work was published in *Cancer Research*, reported, *"Cancer cells demonstrate a 3- to 5-fold increase in glucose uptake compared to healthy cells."*

One of the methods modern medicine uses to detect the origin or spread of cancer is the PET (positron emission tomography) scan. Simply put, cancer patients are injected with radioactive-labeled sugar into their veins, cancer cells absorb the labeled sugar, and this is how cancerous organs are detected. Increased metabolic uptake of sugar locates cancer. Sugar fuels cancer cells. Sugar and cancer "are locked in a death grip," says Dr. Mark Sircus of the International Medical Veritas Association.

Sugar has been called the "white death." An average American is said to consume about 160–200 pounds of sugar a year! Processed foods, cakes, sweets and doughnuts are made up of white sugar, corn syrup and processed flour. Soft drinks, soda and fruit juice are all sugar and chemical additives. All wheat products turn into sugar in the body. Processing sugar for the body is taxing. One molecule of sugar requires more than 50 molecules of magnesium. Due to excessive consumption of sugar, it is suggested that's why there's such a magnesium deficiency in our modern culture.

In our body, all starches and carbohydrates get metabolized down to sugar, or glucose. Sugar destroys the healthy gut flora and immune system. Processed carbohydrates and sugars feed the "bad" bacteria and fungi in the gut flora, helping them grow and proliferate, causing dysbiosis.

Excessive sugar in the body leads to the "rusting" of our organs, blood vessels and brain. Our blood in our arteries that supply fresh oxygen to our heart is supposed to be free-flowing, like water. When too much sugar is consumed, glycation occurs. A sugar molecule pairs up with a protein, and this molecular arrangement alters the protein structure and destroys its function. These high blood-sugar complexes, measured as HgA1C in blood work, damage tissues and organs, including disrupting the transport of blood gases. Blood becomes thick, laced with glycation sugar complexes, and the water becomes like maple syrup. It forms a "traffic jam" in the vessels full of sugar, and blood flow is slow, acidic and damaging to the organs, heart, brain, kidneys, liver and gut. This glycation causes high blood pressure, fatigue and brain fog. Eventually this leads to insulin resistance, and type 2 diabetes, poor immune function, disease and cancer formation. Cancer loves sugar. Sugar is acidic, destroys the gut health and cripples the immune system.

AVOID ALCOHOL!

Herb is the healing of a nation,
alcohol is the destruction.

—Bob Marley

Research has consistently shown that any form of alcohol, such as beer, wine or liquor, increases the risk of cancer. More recently, according to a 2016 literature review in *Addiction*, there is strong evidence that alcohol causes seven cancers and may cause more. According to lead researcher Jennie Conner, from the University of Otago in New Zealand, evidence supports a causal association between alcohol consumption and cancers of the breast, liver, colon, rectum, oropharynx, larynx and esophagus.

Even moderate drinking has shown to increase breast cancer in women. Research shows that compared to women who don't drink alcohol at all, women who drink alcohol three times a week have a 15% increased risk of breast cancer. There is about a 10% increased risk of breast cancer with each additional drink each day!

If someone is actively fighting cancer, they must give up sugar and alcohol, completely. If someone is preventing a recurrence of cancer, they have an occasional drink with food. If someone is trying to prevent ever having cancer, they have alcohol moderately, an eight-ounce glass with food. They have happy balance with regular exercise, sleep and whole, organic plant-based foods.

BECOME ALKALINE!

Water, air and cleanliness are the chief articles
in my pharmacopoeia.

—Napoleon

An acidic body is out of balance. Eating a diet full of processed foods, sugar, alcohol, dairy, excessive red meat, soda and energy drinks, combined with stress, shallow breathing, poor sleep and lack of exercise, are poor habits that promote an acidic environment in the body. An acidic body means a poor immune system with chronic disease and cancer.

Cancer is anaerobic; it does not need oxygen to grow. Most infections, bacterial, viral and fungal, all generate and thrive in an acidic pH environment. Our healthy cells are aerobic; they need oxygen in every cell to thrive, as discussed previously. Cancer thrives in an acidic condition. Cancer cells also give off lactic acid during their anaerobic fermentation of foods to lower the body pH even more and further weaken the body's ability to fight back. Invading bacterial, viral and fungal cells also generates lactic acid to handicap the innate immune response.

The human body requires a blood pH of 7.4 to survive. A more alkaline body means a strong immune system with health and a disease-free state. The lower the body pH (pH 1 being acidic, 7 being neutral, pH 14 being alkaline), the more compromised the body's immune system. It is important to eat more alkaline foods and have alkaline habits. According to Dr. Ragnar Berg, an acclaimed Swedish nutritionist, it is optimal to eat 80% alkaline foods and only 20% acidic foods for daily intake. I would suggest doing the same for habits as well, 80% alkaline habits, 20% acidic habits daily, to keep the immune system optimal.

Alkaline foods are plant-based foods, such as vegetables, fruits, nuts, seeds, grains, and beans. Alkaline habits are exercise, adequate hydration, deep breathing, and taking a probiotic.

Acidic foods and acidic habits need to be minimized. Acidic foods are refined sugars, processed foods, bread, wheat, dairy, animal proteins, soda, coffee and alcohol. Acidic habits are poor sleep, stress, not exercising, smoking, drinking alcohol and anxiety.

Some acidic foods, like lemon, lime, oranges, tomatoes and apple cider vinegar create an "alkaline tide" when they are exposed to our salivary glands or digestive enzymes. This means they turn alkaline and are heavily beneficial to the body's health. This is amazing; the miraculous power of Mother Nature and God, how we are able to convert even nature's acidic foods into healing alkaline pH to combat cancer, infections and disease.

BREATHE OXYGEN!

Long breath, long Life. Short breath, short life.

—Toa saying

Humans are aerobes. This means we require oxygen to survive. We can barely survive without one minute of oxygen. Oxygen is life-preserving. Healthy cells are aerobic; they require oxygen. Cancer cells are anaerobic. They do not require oxygen to grow, and they thrive in acidic conditions. When we shallow breathe, we have less oxygen and more acid in the body. When we deep breathe, we get more oxygen and become more alkaline.

Relearn to take slow, deep breaths all day long. Deep breaths of oxygen increase blood flow, reduce acid, remove toxins and help fight off cancer.

TAKE POWERHOUSE SUPPLEMENTS!

All those vitamins aren't to keep death at bay,
they're to keep deterioration at bay.

—Jeanne Moreau,
French actress, singer, director

Along with eating wholesome food, take antioxidants supplements: resveratrol, quercetin, DIM, NAC, curcumin, vitamin D3, omega-3 fatty oils, S-acytle glutathione, ALA, iodine, and vitamins A, C, E, NAD+ and systemic enzymes.

Scientists are now postulating that some cancers are infection-derived, an estimated 15–20%. It is important to boost our immune system with antioxidants and anti-inflammatory foods and vitamins. Previous fungal, viral and bacterial infections that took host in the human DNA can be expressed later as cancers. Researches are finding most infection-caused cancers are due to viruses and others by bacteria.

Listed Below Are Some Examples:

- Cervical and anogenital cancer—human papillomavirus (HPV)
- Lymphoma—HIV and Epstein-Barr virus
- Liver cancer—hepatitis B and C virus
- Stomach cancer—H. pylori

Research tells us that only 5–10% of all cancers are genetic defects, and the remaining 90–95% are due to environmental and lifestyle factors. That empowers us with a tremendous opportunity to prevent cancer!

CHAPTER 26

Powerful Anti-Cancer Habits

An ounce of prevention is worth a pound of cure.

—Benjamin Franklin

PREVENT AND FIGHT CANCER

These are some powerful methods to help prevent and fight cancer.

1. Be at healthy body weight. Body fat for females should be 16–25% and for males, 8–18%.
2. Balance and optimize your hormones.
3. Cut out refined sugar. Sugar is toxic.
4. Fix gut health. Take a medical-grade probiotic daily.
5. Drink green tea. A daily dose of green tea can help ward off cancer and keep healthy cells from turning cancerous. Its powerful polyphenolic properties are immune stimulants, neutralize free radicals, promote tumor-killing cell rates and inhibit cancer metastasis.
6. Exercise 4 to 5 a week consistently.
7. Sleep 7 to 8 hours a night.

8. Eat organic.

9. Eat a plant-based diet, especially leafy greens, and minimize animal proteins; if eating animal proteins, they should only be grass-fed and pasture-raised meats and dairy products.

10. Breathe deeply.

11. Detox chemical-based makeup, cleaning agents, GMO foods and nitrate-based foods; quit smoking, vaping and chewing tobacco.

12. Minimize or quit alcohol consumption.

13. Take antioxidant supplements—resveratrol, quercetin, DIM, curcumin, NAD+, vitamin D3, omega-3 fatty oils, S-acytle glutathione, ALA, iodine, systemic enzymes and vitamins A, C, and E.

13. Cultivate positive thinking.

PART IV

CELL REGENERATION

CHAPTER 27

Optimizing Telomeres—Stem Cell Preservation and Regeneration

Though nobody can go back and make a new beginning...
Anyone can start over and make a new ending.

—Chico Xavier

THE SCIENCE BEHIND A LONG, HAPPY AND HEALTHY LIFESPAN is continuously emerging. Preserving our DNA and stem cells are crucial for extending life and retaining health. Each person is born with a certain number of adult stem cells. At birth, we have the highest amount of stem cells (EPCs and MSCs). After thirty years old, we start declining in our stem cells and, with major health problems, they decline even more steeply. The rate of division of our stem cells, especially mesenchymal stem cells (MSCs), slows down. MSCs have regenerating properties, are found in every tissue and are attached to blood vessels. They control inflammation and the immune system, stimulate regeneration, and reduce scarring. They maintain our natural repair mechanisms throughout the entire body. Endothelial precursor cells (EPCs) are mostly found in bone marrow and circulate throughout the bloodstream. Dr. Neil Riordan, a scientific leader in stem cell studies, reports that low EPCs are connected to heart attacks, stroke, Alzheimer's disease, high blood pressure, diabetes, sleep apnea, erectile dysfunction, migraines and kidney failure. He reports higher circulating stem cells are important to remain healthy.

Stem cells continually diminish with age. Our lifestyle and hormones determine how quickly we burn through our stem cells. Optimizing each hormone improves our endogenous stem cell production and function. Balanced hormones improve the endothelial lining to help regenerate stem cells and allow for a healthier body, slowing down the aging process and preventing chronic diseases and the depletion of stem cells.

Our DNA is the code of life. It is the template for every cell in the body and makes us unique. DNA is a double helix made up of four base pairs and holds all of our heredity material. DNA must replicate (mitosis) and make copies of itself to carry on life, regenerate and repair. Our DNA is tightly packaged into chromosomes, which are dense threadlike structures. Each chromosome has a protective end cap called a telomere. The human species has 23 pairs of chromosomes. One pair is inherited from the mother and the other pair from the father. The last pair of chromosomes determines our sex; women have XX, and men have XY chromosomes. These chromosomes are located in the nucleus (brain) of every living cell in our body. Each time a cell replicates, it is critical that the new cell has an exact copy of the old DNA. And, each time a cell replicates, a small piece of DNA and telomere is taken off the end of each chromosome. Aging cells lose their DNA repair mechanism, resulting in DNA genetic damage. This can cause cells to replicate and proliferate out of control, turning into cancer cells.

TELOMERES: THE AGING CLOCK OF EVERY CELL!

Telomeres are the tiny end caps of chromosomes. They act like the plastic tips at the end of shoelaces to prevent chromosomes from fraying. They protect the genetic information in the DNA. Every day our

DNA replicates, enduring millions of damaging effects and, amazingly, our cells have powerful built-in methods of self-correcting— TELOMERES! All healthy cells have this DNA gene repair mechanism. Each human cell has 92 telomeres. They are a unique repeat sequence of base pairs, TTAGGG.

As mentioned, DNA must replicate itself precisely and properly for life to carry on. Each time a cell replicates, a small piece of DNA and telomere is taken off. Telomeres are lost in the process of replication, a little at a time. The shorter the telomere gets, the more cellular aging, and it can no longer protect the cell's DNA. Eventually, too much of the telomere is lost and DNA can no longer replicate, leading to cell death. Cell death is called senescence. Also, when telomeres become too short or are depleted, cells stop replicating accurately, and errors occur, called mutations. This DNA damage leads to disease, cancer and a shorter life.

Shortened telomere length correlates with a worsened immune system, brain fog, fatigue, weight gain and an increase in degenerative diseases such as diabetes, heart disease, Alzheimer's and death. A large study from the University of Copenhagen, Demark, followed 19,838 men and women for 19 years. The researchers found that short telomeres increased the risk of heart attacks by 50% and the risk of early death by 25%.

Extended telomere length leads to cell regeneration, increased immune system, hair growth and color, less brain fog and greater youthfulness. Longer telomere length means longer lifespan.

WHAT DAMAGES TELOMERE LENGTH?

Telomeres act as aging clocks for each cell in the body. Shortened telomeres mean premature cellular aging and lead to disease formation. Shortened telomeres are caused by chronic stress, biological aging, not exercising, smoking, obesity, poor sleep and poor nutrition. Free radicals and synthetic compounds damage DNA. Stress has been shown to accelerate the shortening of telomeres.

At the highest level of telomere length, we have 10,000 base pairs at the end of each chromosome. By 25 to 35 years old, we have 7,000–8,000 base pairs left. By 65 years old, we have only 4,800 base pairs left. They shorten with each cell division. Studies show that high levels of stress cause shortening of telomeres. Studies have also shown that women who have been chronically stressed have shortened telomeres and DNA that looked 10 to 15 years older compared to their low-stress counterparts' telomere lengths. Shortened telomeres mean accelerated aging! To properly restore and maintain telomeres is the secret to youthfulness.

WHAT EXTENDS AND PRESERVES TELOMERE LENGTH?

In 2009, three Harvard scientists were awarded the Nobel Prize for discovering how an enzyme called telomerase. Telomerase is an enzyme made in the body that makes telomeres longer. Together, the scientists discovered that turning "on" telomerase reversed aging in mice, especially in their brain cells. Research has shown that the amount of telomerase we make decreases with age, and replacement of telomerase could reverse and even lengthen telomeres. This process would allow cells to live longer, replicate again, and repair old cells like they used to work, thereby, slowing down aging and possibly extending lifespan.

WHAT REGENERATES TELOMERES?

Scientists have found that along with genetics, lifestyle, diet and exercise all play enormous roles in extending telomeres and reversing the aging process. Scientists have found that a healthy diet and nutrition will prevent telomere shortening and actually lead to telomere lengthening. Dr. Mark Tarnopolsky, a professor and researcher focused on mitochondria, found that exercise increases levels of a molecule that protects telomeres and prevents their shortening. He showed in his research that exercise slowed down aging at the cellular, telomere level. He suggested that by exercising regularly, you can slow down the speed of aging and can increase your lifespan by five years. Another study found that a three-month training program of just walking at moderate intensity increased circulating endothelial precursor cells (EPC) stem cells by 120%.

WHAT CAN YOU DO TO REGENERATE YOUR TELOMERES?

- Exercise regularly
- Drink green tea
- Breath properly
- Balance your hormones
- Keep your brain active, read books
- Eat grapes, blueberries and gogi berries
- Take supplements: vitamins C, E, A, D3, omega-3, polyphenols, resveratrol, folate and astragalus extract. These have shown to up-regulate telomerase and increase telomere length.

We have a choice every single day to preserve our stem cells or destroy them. Eating green leafy vegetables and nuts, sleep, exercise, sex, breathing and laughter (release of endorphins) also have shown to increase telomere length.

CHAPTER 28

Sirtuins—The Longevity Genes!

Natural forces within us are the true healers of disease.

—Hippocrates

WHAT ARE SIRTUINS?

Sirtuins are a family of genes that manage the body's defenses during hard and stressful times. They are also known as the housekeeping genes. Mammals have seven sirtuin proteins designated SIRT-1 to SIRT-7. Sirtuins are master regulators of our survival instinct and how we respond to stress in order to sustain our health and prolong our life. Their primary role is to help the body "get fired up for survival mode!" They promote survival and stress resistance and, for this, are deemed the "longevity genes."

Sirtuins are in charge of figuring out which cells survive, decreasing inflammation, increasing fat metabolism and determining insulin resistance. They get us through times we thought we'd never endure and keep us surviving. They determine our aging by stress-induced apoptosis (cell death) and cell defense. To protect the body against cancer and disease, they induce autophagy, a natural, regulated mechanism to eliminate or recycle damaged cells. They play a major role in selective gene expression, turning on and off what we need to sustain the body's survival. They're involved in DNA repair and energy metabolism. They get the body revved up for whatever it takes to survive. It's amazing how the body has its own amazing capacity to sustain longevity!

Scientists are still researching and learning about sirtuins; the following are some known functions:

- SIRT1 is known to regulate brain plasticity and memory formation.
- SIRT3–5 are known as mitochondrial sirtuin, renewing and preserving mitochondria, and preventing oxidation.
- SiRT6 regulates the telomere length.

HOW DO WE PRESERVE AND BOOST OUR SIRTUINS?

They are preserved and increased by eating "sirtfoods," exercising, fasting and caloric restriction. Sirtuins are decreased by a high-fat diet. There are actually "sirtfoods" that increase and activate our sirtuins! Mother Nature has an extraordinary way of preserving life. Just eating more "sirtfoods" easily extends life naturally. Other methods of increasing our sirtuin activity are calorie restriction (CR) eating habits, taking resveratrol, and NAD+.

WHAT ARE SOME "SIRTFOODS"?

Sirtfoods include green tea, kale, olives, omega-3 fish oils, onions, curcumin, parsley, organic tofu, miso soup, citrus fruits, apples, extra virgin olive oil, dark chocolate, black currants and capers.

CALORIE RESTRICTION (CR) ENHANCES LIFESPAN

About 80 years ago, scientists discovered the benefits of calorie restriction (CR). It is the only proven method for life extension. It acts as a life stressor and activates sirtuin genes because the body realizes food scarcity and revs up its defensive responses to boost survival. When sirtuins "up-regulate" due to calorie restriction, they respond by enacting cellular repair, energy production, programmed cell death and DNA repair. CR means reducing your calorie intake by 30–40% and avoiding malnutrition by taking in plenty of nutrient-rich organic whole foods and hydrating well.

In animal studies, those that were calorie-restricted lived longer and were healthier than their counterparts. In studies, CR increased life expectancy by over 30%! This is because CR improves insulin sensitivity, improves carbohydrate metabolism and increases mitochondrial function, and so helps fight obesity, inflammation and diabetes by burning stored fats and sugars, and releasing abundant energy.

In 2014, after studying the Japanese Okinawan diet, the University of Wisconsin did their own study. Okinawans follow a modest calorie restriction diet, limiting calories by only 11%, and have averaged the longest recorded life spans in the world! They experience less heart disease, diabetes, cancer and Alzheimer's disease. The University of Washington did their CR study on adult monkeys, only mildly calorie-restricting them. They found that the animals with a regular diet had a 2.9 times greater rate of death from age-related causes than the calorie-restricted animals. This also showed that starting a CR diet at any point in life still provides significant benefits. CR diet, quercetin, resveratrol and NAD+ all increase sirtuin activity.

CR is doing done best by following the three-fourths rule. Only eat three-fourths of your meal.

BENEFITS OF CALORIE RESTRICTION (CR)

Following are benefits of following a calorie restriction diet.

- Activates sirtuin genes
- Restores and extends telomere length
- Lowers body fat
- Bolsters insulin sensitivity
- Reduces inflammation, especially neurotoxins
- Increases HGH release
- Increases mitochondrial function
- Improves energy

BENEFITS OF NAD+

Following are benefits of NAD+:

- Neuro-protective (helps fight Alzheimer's and Parkinson's diseases)
- Cardio-protective
- Restores and supports mitochondria
- Helps improve metabolism
- Improves blood flow
- Increases muscle endurance and growth; combats sarcopenia (muscle wasting) in the elderly
- Increases insulin sensitivity
- Increases energy production
- Repairs DNA
- Maintains and protects healthy DNA
- Activates sirtuins
- Restores brain plasticity

BENEFITS OF RESVERATROL

Following are benefits of resveratrol:

- A plant chemical found in grape skin, blueberries, raspberries and mulberries and peanuts that mimic CR benefits
- Increases sirtuin activity, specifically SIRT1 to SIRT3
- Provides cancer protection
- Is cardio-protective and vasculo-protective, so protects against heart disease
- Is an actively strong antioxidant, down-regulates inflammation
- Increases cell autophagy to help defend body from disease
- Has anti-cancer properties, suppresses new cancer growth
- "Trans" is the active form, so use trans-resveratrol when getting the supplement.

The goal of health is to keep the body in a thriving state of being, to REGENERATE! We have learned that restoring and balancing hormones, getting quality nutrition, proper breathing, restorative sleep, consistent exercise and having a positive mindset can do this.

Final Thoughts

Our lives are the sum of the choices we make.
—Albert Camus

LIFE IS A BALANCE EVERY DAY. EVERYTHING WE DO regenerates or degenerates our health. Think about that. *You* have a choice every single day to pause aging and regenerate your life. The goal isn't to feel normal—it's to feel *extraordinary!* Here are some powerful thoughts to keep in mind to Grow Younger and keep Regenerating!

1. Life is magical. Don't ever stop believing in miracles.
2. Eat organic, plant-based foods, as much as possible.
3. Balance and restore your hormones.
4. Exercise 4 to 5 times a week.
5. Eat a huge handful of raw mixed nuts every day.
6. Forgive.
7. BREATHE. Breathe deeply.
8. Love and laughter are the tonics of life.
9. Drink green tea 2 to 3 times a day.
10. Take resveratrol, vitamin D3 and curcumin every day.

11. Be kind. Give, give, give, and learn to receive.

12. Sugar is toxic; it feeds cancer.

13. Start the morning drinking alkaline water with fresh lemon.

14. Eat slowly and only eat three-fourths of your food.

15. Sleep is precious; get 7 to 8 hours.

16. Pray... Live in gratitude every single day.

17. Give hugs and kisses to loved ones every day.

18. Orgasms keep you forever young.

19. Real Wealth = Health + Longevity (more Time for Being and Loving)

20. Treat your body like a temple. Don't pollute it.

21. Become an ETERNAL OPTIMIST!

Our prime purpose in this life is to help others.
And if you can't help them, at least don't hurt them.

—Dalai Lama

References

Chapter 2

Anderson V, et al. Estrogen, cognition and woman's risk of Alzheimer's disease. *Am J Med.* 1997;103(3A):11S–18S.

Arver S, et al. Improvement of sexual function in testosterone deficient men treated for 1 year with a permeation enhanced testosterone transdermal system. *J Urol* 1996;155:1604–1608.

Bera, V. Million Women Study Collaborators. Breast cancer and hormone-replacement therapy in the Million Women Study. *Lancet* 2003;362:419–427.

Boosma D, Paoletti, J. A review of current research on the effects of progesterone. *Int J Pharm Compd* 2002;6:245–248.

Braga-Basaria M. Metabolic syndrome in men with prostate cancer undergoing longterm androgen-deprivation therapy. *J Clin Oncol.* 2006;24(24):3979–3983.

Braverman E. *Younger You: Unlock the Hidden Power of Your Brain to Look and Feel 15 Years Younger*, New York, NY: McGraw-Hill Companies; 2007.

Braverman LE, Utiger RD, eds. *Werner & Ingbar's The Thyroid: A Fundamental and Clinical Text*, Sixth Ed. New York, NY: JB Lippincott; 1981.

Brownstein D. *Iodine: Why You Need It, Why You Can't Live Without It*, 4th Ed. Bloomfield Hills, MI: Medical Alternative Press; 2009.

Brownstein D. *The Miracle of Natural Hormones*. Bloomfield Hills, MI: Medical Alternative Press; 2003.

Bunevicius R, et al. Effects of thyroxine as compared with thyroxine plus triiodothyroxine in patients with hypothyroidism *N Engl J Med* 1999;340:424–429.

Bussiere JR, et al. Androgen deprivation impairs memory in older men. *Behav Neurosci* 2005;119–143.

Canonico M, et al., Hormone therapy and venous thromboembolism among postmenopausal women. Impact of the route of estrogen administration and progestogens: The ESTHER study. *Circulation* 2007;115:840–845.

Chang KJ, et al. Influences of percutaneous administration of estradiol and progesterone on human breast epithelial cell cycle in vivo. *Amer Soc Reprod Med* 1995;63(4):785–791.

Chetkowski R, et al. Biological effects of transdermal estradiol, *N Engl J Med* 1986;314:1615–1620.

Christianson A. How Much Iodine Do You Need For Thyroid Disease? Web site: http://drchristianson.com/how-much-iodine-do-you-need-for-thyroid-disease/. Accessed October 11, 2018.

Cohen PG. Diabetes mellitus is associated with subnormal levels of free testosterone in men. *Brit J Urol* 2006;97(3):652–653.

Cowan LD, et al. Breast cancer incidence in women with a history of progesterone deficiency. *Am J Epidemiol* 1981;114:209–217.

Dai WS, et al. Relationship between plasma high-density lipoprotein cholesterol and sex hormone concentrations in men. *Am J Cardiol* 1984;53:1259–1263.

Davis SR, et al. Testosterone enhances estradiol's effect on postmenopausal bone density and sexuality. *Maturitas.* 1995;21(3):227–236.

Ding E, et al. Sex differences of endogenous sex hormones and risk of type 2 diabetes: a systemic review and a meta-analysis. *JAMA* 2006;295:1288–1299.

Dordona P, et al. Update: hypogonadotropic hypogonadism in type 2 diabetes and obesity. *J Clin Endocrinol Met* 2011;96(9):2643.

Fitspatrick LA, Pace C, Wiita B. Comparison of regimens containing oral micronized progesterone or medroxyprogesterone acetate on quality of life in postmenopausal women: A cross-sectional survey. *J Womens Health Gend Based Med* 2000;9(4):381–387.

Fournier A, et al. Breast cancer risk in relation to different types of hormone replacement therapy in the E3N-EPIC cohort. *Int J Cancer.* 2005;114:448–454.

Godsland IF. Effects of postmenopausal hormonal replacement therapy on lipid, lipoprotein, and apolipoprotein (a) concentrations: Analysis of studies published from 1974–2000. *Fertil Steril.* 2001;75(5):898–915.

Hertoghe T. *The Hormone Handbook,* London: International Medical Books: 2006.

Holtorf K. The bioidentical hormone debate: Are bioidentical hormones (estradiol, estriol, and progesterone) safer or more efficacious than commonly used synthetic versions in hormone replacement therapy? *Postgrad Med.* 2009;January:121.

Information: http://www.cdc.gov/women/lcod.htm

Klatz R., Goldman, R. *The Official Anti-Aging Revolution: Stop the Clock, Time is on Your Side, For a Younger, Stronger, Happier You,* Fourth Edition, North Bergen, NJ: Basic Health Publications; 2007.

Klein I, et al. "Thyroid hormone and the cardiovascular system, *New Engl J Med* 2002;344:501–509.

Kutty KM, et al. Serum lipids in hypothyroidism: a re-evaluation. *J Clin Endo Metab* 1978;46:55–56.

Laaksonen D, et al. Testosterone and sex hormone-binding globulin predict the metabolic syndrome and diabetes in middle-aged men. *Diabetes Care* 2004;27:1037–1041.

Lee JR. *What Your Doctor May Not Tell You About Breast Cancer* New York, NY: Warner Books; 2003.

Lee JR. *What Your Doctor May Not Tell You About Menopause.* New York, NY: Warner Books; 1996.

Lee JR. *What Your Doctor May Not Tell You About Perimenopause.* New York, NY: Warner Books; 1999.

Leonetti HB, Longo S, Anasti JN. Transdermal progesterone cream for vasomotor symptoms and postmenopausal bone loss. *Obstet Gynecol* 1999;94(2):225–228.

Lichten EM. *Textbook of Bio-Identical Hormones.* Michigan: Foundation for Anti-Aging Reseach; 2007.

Life Extension Magazine. Bioidentical hormones: Why are they still controversial? Web site: http://www.lifeextension.com/magazine/2009/10/Bioidentical-Hormones. October, 2009. Accessed 10/11/2018.

Liverman C, Blazer D, eds. *Testosterone and Aging: Clinical Research Directions*. Washington, DC: The National Academies Press; 2004.

Mikhail N. Does testosterone have a role in erectile function? *Amer J of Med*. 2006; 119(5):373–82.

Miner MM, et al., Testosterone ad ageing: what have we learned since the institute of medicine report and what lies ahead? *Int J Clin Pract*. 2007 Apr;61(4):622–32.

Morgentaler A. Testosterone and prostate cancer: an historical perspective on a modern myth. *Eur Urol* 2006;50(5):895–897.

Morgentaler A. Testosterone replacement therapy and prostate risks: where's the beef? *Can J Urol* 2006 Feb;13(1):40–43.

Morgentaler A. Testosterone therapy for men at risk for or with a history of prostate cancer. *Curr Treat Options Oncol* 2006;7(5):363–369.

Morgentaler, A, et al., Prevalence of prostate cancer among hypogonadal men with prostate-specific antigen levels of 4.0 ng/mL or less. *Curr Ther Res Clin Exp* 2006 Dec;68(6):1263–1266.

Nathorst-Boos J. Treatment with percutaneous testosterone gel in postmenopausal women with decreased libido-effects on sexuality and psychological general well-being. *Maturitas*. 2006;53(1):11–18.

Nike E, et al. Estrogens as antioxidants. *Methods Enczymol*. 1990;186:330.

Phillips GB, Pinkernell BH, Jing TY. The association of hypotestosteronemia with coronary artery disease in men. *Arterioscler Thromb* 1994;14:701–706.

Pope HG, Jr., et al. Testosterone gel supplementation for men with refractory depression: a randomized, placebo-controlled trial. *Am J Psychiatry* 2003;160:105–111.

Raz P, Stamm WE. A controlled trial of intravaginal estriol in postmenopausal women with recurrent urinary tract infection. *N Engl J Med* 1993;329(11):753–756.

Rossouw JE, et al. Risks and benefits of estrogen plus progestin in healthy postmenopausal women: Principle results from the Women's Health Initiative randomized controlled trial. *JAMA* 2002;288:321–333.

Rothenberg R, Becker K, Hart K. *Forever Ageless: Advanced Edition.* Encinitas, CA: California Healthspan Institute; 2007.

Rylance PB, Brincat M. Natural progesterone and antihypertensive action. *Br Med J* 1985;290:13.

Saad F, et al. Effects of testosterone on erectile function; implications for the therapy of erectile dysfunction. *Br J Urol* Epub 2007 Feb 15.

Schatzl G, et al. High-grade prostate cancer is associated with low serum testosterone levels. *Prostate* 2001;47:52–58.

Shippen E. *The Testosterone Syndrome.* Lanham, MD: M. Evans & Co; 1999.

Shumaker SA, et al. Estrogen plus progestin and the incidence of dementia and mild cognitive impairment in postmenopausal women: The Women's Health Initiative Memory Study: A randomized controlled trial. *JAMA* 2003;289:2651–2662.

Sinatra S. *The Sinatra Solution.* North Bergen, NJ: Basic Health; 2005.

Smith P. *What You Must Know About Women's Hormones: Your Guide to Natural Hormone Treatments For PMS, Menopause, Osteoporosis, PCOS, and More.* Garden City Park, NY: Square One Publishers; 2010.

Sourrander L, et al. Cardiovascular and cancer morbidity and mortality and sudden cardiac death in postmenopausal women on estrogen replacement therapy (ERT), *Lancet* 1998 Dec 19–26;352(9145):1965–1969.

Steidle CP. New advances in the treatment of hypogonadism in the aging male. *Review Urology.* 2003;5 Supp 1:S34–S40.

Stephenson K, et al. Topical progesterone cream does not increase thrombotic and inflammatory factors in postmenopausal women. *Blood* 2004;104:5318.

Sullivan JM, et al. Estrogen replacement and coronary disease. Effects on survival in postmenopausal women. *Arch Intern Med* 1990 Dec;150(12):2557–2562.

Tenover JL. Testosterone and the aging male. *J Androl* 1997;18:103–106.

Travison TG, et al. A population-level decline in serum testosterone levels in American men. *J Clin Endocrinol Metab* 2007;92:196–202.

Utian W. NAMS releases updated positions statement on HT. *OB-GYN News* 2007;42(4):1.

Vermeulen A. Clinical review 24: Androgens in the aging male. *J Clin Endocrinol Metab* 1991;73:221–224.

Waters R. Estrogen to prevent Alzheimer's. *Health* 1997;11(1):1940–1942.

West J. *Prevent, Survive, Thrive: Every Women's Guide to Optimal Breast Care.* Houston, TX: BenBella Books; 2016.

Wilson JL, *Adrenal Fatigue: The 21st Century Stress Syndrome.* Petaluma, CA; Smart Publications; 2001.

Winkler U, Effects of androgens on homeostasis. *Maturitas.* 1996;24:147–155.

Winters, S. Current status of testosterone replacement therapy in men. *Arch Fam Med* 1999;8:259–263.

Wiren S, et al. Androgens and prostate cancer risks: a prospective study. *Prostate* 2007;67:1230–1237.

Women and heart disease fact sheet/data & statistics/DHDSP/CDC. Web site: https://www.cdc.gov/dhdsp/data_statistics/fact_sheets/fs_women_heart.htm

Wood C, et al. Effect of estradiol with micronized progesterone or medroxyprogesterone acetate on risk markers for breast cancer in postmenopausal monkeys. *Breast Cancer Res Treat* 2007;101:125–134.

Wright JV, Lenard, L. *Stay Young & Sexy with Bio-Identical Hormone Replacement* North Haledon, NJ: Smart Publications; 2010.

Yen-Ping Ho J, et al. Differential effects of oral conjugated equine estrogens and transdermal estrogen on atherosclerotic vascular disease (ASVD) risk markers and endothelial function in healthy postmenopausal women. *Hum Reprod.* 2006;21(10):2715–2720.

Yonker J, et al. Verified hormone therapy improves episodic memory performance in healthy postmenopausal women. *Neuropsychol Dev Cogn B Aging Neuropsychol Cogn.* 2006;13;291–307.

Chapter 9

Biok J. *Cancer and Natural Medicine.* Oregon: Oregon Medical Press; 1995.

Campbell-McBride N. *GAPS: Gut and Psychology Syndrome, Natural treatment for Dyspraxia, Autism, ADD, Dyslexia, ADHD, Depression, Schizophrenia.* Norfolk, UK: Medinform; 2012.

Cummings JH, Macfarlane GT. Colonic microflora: Nutrition and health. *Nutrition* 1997;21(6):357–365.

Cunningham-Rundles S, et al. Probiotics and immune response. *Am J Gastroenterol* 1997;93 (suppl):89–99.

Finegold SM, Sutter VL, Mathisen GE, Normal indigenous intestinal flora. In: Hentges DJ, ed. *Human Intestinal Flora in Health and Disease.* London, UK: Academic Press; 1983:3–31.

Fraser Gary. *Diet, Life Expectancy, and Chronic Disease: Studies of Seventh-day Adventists and Other Vegetarians* Oxford, UK: Oxford University Press; 2003.

Fuhrman J. *Eat to Live: The Amazing Nutrient-Rich Program for Fast and Sustained Weight Loss,* Revised edition. Boston, MA: Little, Brown and Company; 2011.

Gershon M. *The Second Brain: The Scientific Basis of Gut Instinct and a Groundbreaking New Understanding of Nervous Disorders of the Stomach and Intestines.* New York, NY: HarperCollins; 1998.

Life Extension. Unique probiotic targets cardiovascular disease. *Life Extension Magazine.* 2014;October:45–52.

Mokdad AH, et al. The spread of the obesity epidemic in the United States, 1991–1998. *JAMA* 1999;282(16):1519–1522.

Mondot S, de Wouters T, Dore J, Lepage P. The human gut microbiome and its dysfunction. *Dig Dis* 2013;31(3–4):278–285.

Perlmutter D. *Brain Grain: The Surprising Truth About Wheat, Carbs, and Sugar–Your Brain's Silent Killers.* Boston, MA: Little, Brown and Company; 2013.

Singh P.N, Sabate J, Fraser G. Does low meat consumption increase life expectancy in humans? *Am J Clinl Nut* 2003;Sept:526S–532S.

Wang Y, et al. Will all Americans become overweight or obese? Estimating the progression and cost of the US obesity epidemic. *Obesity* 2008, Oct;16(10):2323–2330.

Yang CS, Wang ZY. Tea and cancer. *J. Natl Cancer Inst* 1993;85:1038.

Chapter 11

Where are GMOs grown and banned? #GMOFAQ. GMO.geneticliteracyprogect.org. Web site: https://www.gmo.geneticliteracyproject.org/FAQ/where-are-gmos-grown-and-banned/

Chapter 12

Everything you should know about manuka honey.
  Web site: http://www.healthline.com/healthy/manuka-honey

Geertsen L. How to use Himalayan sea salt. Web site:
  http://www.empoweredsustenance.com/himalayan-salt-benefits/.
  Accessed November 13, 2018.

Gunnars K. Ten proven benefits of green tea. Web site:
  https://www.healthline.com/nutrition/top-10-evidence-based-health-
  benefits-of-green-tea#section7. Accessed November 13, 2018.

Hertoghe T. *Textbook of Nutrient Therapy*. International Medical Books:
  Luxemburg. 2011.

Life Extension. *Disease Prevention and Treatment*. Fort Lauderdale, FL: Life
  Extension; 2003.

Medical College of Georgia. Green tea linked to skin cell regeneration.
  Web site: https://www.sciencedaily.com/
  releases/2003/04/030425071800.htm. Accessed November 13, 2018.

Middleton, Jr. E, Harbone JB, Beretz A. *Plant Flavonoids in Biology and
  Medicine* II. Wilmington, DE: Liss; 1988.

Percent of adults age 20 years and over with overweight, including
  obesity: 70.7% (2013–2014). Web site: http://www.cdc.gov/
  nchs/fastats/obesity-overweight.htm

Perricone N. *The Perricone Prescription*. Boston, MA: HarperCollins; 2002.

Stanway P. *The Miracle of Apple Cider Vinegar*. New York, NY: Metro Books;
  2012.

Chapter 15

Anderson M. The best anti-aging workout you can do. Web site:
  https://www.shape.com/fitness/tips/best-anti-aging-workout-
  benefits-exercise. Accessed November 13,2018.

Colditz GA, Cannuscio CC, Frazier AL. Physical activity and reduced risk
  of colon cancer: implicatians for prevention. *Cancer Causes Control*.
  1997;8:649–667.

Durk R, et al. Gut microbiota composition is related to cardiorespiratory
  fitness in healthy young adults. *Int J Sport Nut Exerc Metab*.
  2018;July: 1–15.

Oaklander M. The new science of exercise. http://www.time.com/4475628/the -new-science-of -exercise/. Accessed November 13,2018.

San Francisco State University. Healthier hearts equal healthier guts: Study finds gut microbiome related to cardiovascular fitness. *ScienceDaily*. Web site: https://www.sciencedaily.com/releases/2018/07/180711131148.htm. Accessed November 13, 2018.

Skelly L, et al. Human muscle fiber-specific responses of mitochondrial fusion proteins to sprint intervals and moderate-intensity continuous training. *Med Sci Sports Exerc*. 2018;May, 50:149.

Strength training may strengthen life span. Worldhealth.net. Anti-Aging News. http://worldhealth.net/news/strenth-training-may-strenghthen-life-span

Urban RJ, et al. Testosterone administration to elderly men increases skeletal muscle strength and protein systhesis. *Am J Physiol*. 1995;269:E820–E826.

Chapter 16

Aldabai,L, Bahammam AS. Metabolic, endocrine, and immune consequences of sleep deprivation. *Open Respir Med J*. 2011;5:31–43.

Estima S. Sleep your way to the top. Medium. June 12, 2018. https://medium.com/s/story/sleep-your-way-to-the-top-debf3fd15c6

Evening use of light-emitting eReaders negatively affects sleep, circadian timing, and next-morning alertness. https://www.ncbi.nlm.nih.gov/pubmed/25535358

Chapter 17

Breast Cancer Prevention Partners.Timing of exposure. www.safecosmetics.org/get -the-facts/healthandscience/timing-of-exposure/. Accessed November 13, 2018.

Ellithorpe E, Settineri R, Barwick D. *Detox outside the box: Living healthier, better, and longer with the newest chelation therapy*. Irvine, CA: Sierra Publications, 2008.

Page A. 10 Houseplants that detox your home.
Web site: https://www.healthcentral.com/slideshow/
10-houseplants-detox-your-home. Accessed November 13, 2018.

Sughrue K. Phthalates: Are they safe? Web site:
https://www.cbsnews.com/news/phthalates-are-they-safe/. Accessed
November 13,2018.

Chapter 18

Anglin RE, et al. Vitamin D Deficiency and Depression in Adults: Systemic
Review and Meta-analysis. *British Journal of Psychiatry.* 2013;202:100–
107.

Annweiler C, et al. Higher vitamin D dietary intake is associated with
lower risk of alzheimer's disease: A 7-year follow-up, *J Gerontol A Bio
Sci Med Sci* 2012;Nov 67 11:1205–1211.

Gaby A, Wright J, Barz F, Chester R, Constantine G, Thomopson L. *The
Natural Pharmacy*, Third Edition. New York, NY: Crown; 2006.

Hertoghe T. *Textbook of Nutrient Therapy.* International Medical Books;
2011.

Kidd PM. PS (PhosphatidylSerine) *nature's brain booster: A vital lipid
nutrient for memory mood and stress*, 2nd Edition. St. George, Utah: Total
Health Communications; 2007.

Klatz R, Goldman R. *The official anti-aging revolution: Stop the clock, time is
on your side, for a younger, stronger, happier you*, Fourth Edition.
Nashville, TN: Basic Health Publications; 2007.

Lomaestro BM, Malone M. Glutathione in health and disease:
pharmacotherapeutic issues. *Ann Pharmacother*. 1995;Dec,
29(12):1263–1273.

Lopez DA, Williams RM, Miehlke K. *Enzymes: The Fountain of Life.*
Charleston, SC: The Neville Press; 1994.

MacWilliam L. *NutriSearch comparative guide to nutritional supplements for
the americas*, Sixth Edition. Kelowna, Canada: Northern Dimensions;
2017.

MacWilliam, L., *NutriSearch comparative guide to nutritional supplements*,
Fifth Edition. Kelowna, Canada: Northern Dimensions; 2014.

Michael Holick MD. *The vitamin D solution: A 3-step strategy to cure our most common health problems* New York, NY: Hudson Street Press; 2010.

Packer L, et al. Neuroprotection by the metabolic antioxidant alpha-lipoic acid. *Free Radic Biol Med.* 1997;22, (1–2): 359–378.

Pershadsingh HA. Alpha-lipoic acid: physiologic mechanisms and indications for the treatment of metabolic syndrome. *Expert Opin Investig Drugs.* 2007;Mar;16(3):291–302.

Ravidran J, Prasad S, Aggarwal BB. Curcumin and cancer cells: how many ways can curry kill tumor cells selectively? *AAPS J.* 2009;Sept;11(3):495–510.

Sun AY, et al. Botanical phenolics and brain health. *Neuromolecular Med.* 2008;10(4):259–274.

Chapter 19

Davey SG, Frankel S, Yarnell J. Sex and death: Are they related? Findings from the Cearphilly cohort study. *Brit Med J.* 1997;315:1641–1645.

New Cigna Study Reveals Loneliness at Epidemic Levels in America. https://www.cigna.com/newsroom/news-releases/2018/new-cigna-study-reveals-lonliness-at-epidemic-levels-in-america

Orgasm and Longevity/ Life enhancement products. http://www.life-enhancement.com/magazine/article/239-orgasm-and-longevity

Waldinger R. What makes a good life? Lessons from the longest study on happiness. Web site: https://www.ted.com/talks/robert_waldinger_what_makes_a_good_life_lessons_from_the_longest_study_on_happiness. Accessed November 13, 2018.

Chapter 20

Harvard Health Medical School. Optimism and your health. Web site: https://www.health.harvard.edu/heart-health/optimism-and-your-health. Accessed November 13,2018.

Marano HE. The benefits of laughter. Web site: https://www.psychologytoday.com/us/articles/200304/the-benefits-laughter. Accessed November 13, 2018.

Men's Health. The five health benefits of being an optimist. Web site: https://www.menshealth.com/health/g19545491/benefits-being-a-optimist/. Accessed November 13, 2018.

Chapter 21

Breathing Exercise: Three to try / 4-7-8 breath / Andrew Weil, M.D. https://www.drweil.com/health-wellness/body-mind-spirit/ stess-anxiety/breathing-three-exercises/1/

Chang L. Eustress vs. Distress. Web site: https://www.mindfulnessmuse.com/stress-reduction/eustress-vs-distress. Accessed November 13, 2018.

Weil A. *Healthy Aging: A Lifelong Guide to Your Physical and Spiritual Well-Being.* Toronto, Canada: Knopf; 2005.

Chapter 22

Koenig H. *Is Religion Good for Your Health? The Effects of Religion on Physical and Mental Health.* Milton Park, UK: The Haworth Pastoral Press; 1997.

Newsmax Media. 47 Health Benefits of Prayer. Web site: http://fgbt.org/Health-tips/47-health-benefits-of-prayer.html. Accessed November 18,2018.

Chapter 24

Demetrakopoulos, GE, Brennan ME. Tumoricidial potential of nutritional manipulations. *Cancer Res.* 1982;42:756S.

Gullino PM. Glucose consumption by transplanted tumors in vivo. *Cancer Res.* 1967;27:1031.

Quillin P. *Beating cancer with nutrition: Optimal nutrition can improve outcome in medically-treated cancer patients,* Revised edition. Nutrition Times Press; Carlsbad, CA; 2005.

The Guardian. Alcohol is a direct cause of seven forms of cancer. Web site: https://www.theguardian.com/society/2016/jul/22/alcohol-direct-cause-seven-forms-of-cancer-study. Accessed November 13, 2018.

Wheeler RB.The Alcohol-Breast Cancer Connection. Web site: https://www.everydayhealth.com/breast-cancer/preventing/alcohol-use.aspx. Accessed November 13, 2018.

Chapter 25

Anand P, et al. Cancer is a preventable disease that requires major lifestyle changes. *Pharm Res.* 2008;Sept; 25(9):2097–2116.

Massetti GM, Dietz WH, Richardson LC. Excessive weight gain, obesity, and cancer opportunities for clinical intervention [published online October 3, 2017]. *JAMA.* doi:10.1001/jama.2017.15519.

Zheng Y, Met al. Associations of weight gain from early to middle adulthood with major health outcomes later in life. *JAMA.* 2017;318(3):255–269.

Chapter 27

Are Telomeres the Key to Aging and Cancer. https://www.learn.genetics.utah.edu/content/basics/telomeres/

Barja G, Herrero A. Oxidative damage to mitochondrial DNA is inversely related to maximum life span in the heart and brain of mammals. *FASEB J.* 2000;14(2):312–318.

Blackburn EH, et al. Telomeres and telomerase: The path from maize. Tetrahymena and yeast to human cancer and aging. *Nature Med* 2006;12:1133–1138.

Hill JM, et al. Circulating endothelial progenitor cells, vascular function, and cardiovascular risk. *N Engl J Med.* 2003;Feb 13;348(7):593–600.

O'Connor C. Telomeres of Human Chromosomes. *Nature Ed.* 2008;1(1):166.

Riordan N. *Stem Cell Therapy: A Rising Tide, How Stem Cells are Disrupting Medicine and Transforming Lives.* Panama City, Panama; printed in the USA; 2017.

Vega LR, et al. Getting to the end: Telomerase access in yeast and humans. *Nature Rev Molec Cell Biol.* 2003;4:948–959.

Chapter 28

Baur JA, et al. Resveratrol improves health and survival of mice on a high-calorie diet. *Nature* 2006;Nov 16, 444(7117):337–342.

Das A, et al. Impairment of an Endothelial NAD+-H2S Signaling Network is a Reversible Cause of Vascular Aging [published online]. *Cell.* 2018;173:74–89. https://www.doi.org/10.1016/j.cell.2018.02.008.

de la Lastra CA, Villegas I. Resveratrol as an anti-inflammatory and anti-aging agent: mechanisms and clinical implications. *Mol Nutr Food Res.* 2005;May;49(5):405–430.

Fresco P, Borges F, Diniz C, Marques MP. New insights on the anticancer properties of dietary polyphenols. *Med Res Rev.* 2006;Nov;26(6):747–766.

Life Extension, Calorie Restriction Extends Life and Protects Against Age-Related Disease. *Life Extension Magazine.* 2014;Sept:37–39.

Life Extension. New Reason to Avoid Stress. *Life Extension Magazine.* 2012;June:71–79.

Life Extension. Nicotinamide Riboside Sharpens Cognition and Reduces Alzheimer's Risk. *Life Extension Magazine.* 2018;May:63–66.

Mills KF, et al. Long-term administration of nicotinamide mononucleotide mitigates age-associated physiological decline in mice. *Cell Metab.* 2016. PMID 28068222.

Rickman AD, et al. The CALERIE Study: design and methods of an innovative 25% calorie restriction intervention. *Contemp Clin Trials.* 2011;32(6):874–881.

Shoba B, et al. Functions of sirtuins in biological tissues. *The Anatomical Record.* 2009;292:536–543.

Sirtfood Diet. Top 20 Sirtfoods. Web site: https://www.sirtfooddiet.net/articles/top-sirtfoods. Accessed November 13, 2018.

Stefani M, et al. The effect of resveratrol on a cell model of human aging. *Ann N Y Acad Sci.* 2007;Oct;1114:407–418.

Wilson A. Top ten sirtuin foods for good health. Web site: https://www.inner-light-in.com/2015/05/top-ten-sirtuin. Accessed November 13,2018.

Wolf NS, Penn PE, Jiang D, Fei RG, Pendergrass WR. Calorie restriction: conservation of in vivo cellular replicative capacity accompanies life-span extension in mice. *Exp Cell Res.* 1995;Apr;217(2):317–323.

Index

About the Author

GOWRI REDDY ROCCO, M.D., M.S., is double board-certified in Family Medicine and in Regenerative, Anti-Aging and Functional Medicine. She has been practicing medicine for almost 20 years and is co-founder and president of Optimum Wellness & Longevity in Corona, California. Dr. Gowri has a successful practice alongside her husband and is a proud mother of three wonderful children.

Dr. Gowri was born in Tirupati, South India. She was six years old when she moved to the United States with her parents, brother and sister. She grew up in Michigan, fully enjoying and loving the great outdoors. Dr. Gowri is passionate about incorporating eastern culture and medicine with her practice of western medicine, infusing it into her practice to heal her patients, loved ones, and herself.

Dr. Gowri loves spending her time with her family at the beach, walking barefoot on sand and grass, loves to cook and is passionate about eating culinary foods, loves fashion, loves hiking, pilates, resistance training, dancing, reading, journaling, traveling, and going on walks and riding bikes with her kids. She treasures her time with her family and friends.

Dr. Gowri is also passionate about her family's philanthropic missionary work—building a hospital in southern India—which her father started in honor of her sister Padma Reddy. This hospital, the Sri Venkateswara Psychiatric Foundation, nested within the family ashram, provides free mental health services to the needy and poverty-stricken. A portion of the proceeds from this book will be donated to support this family cause.

To learn more about Dr. Gowri Reddy Rocco, or her practice, Optimum Wellness & Longevity, go to DrGowri.com or OptimumWL.com.

Blessings of Health and Happiness!

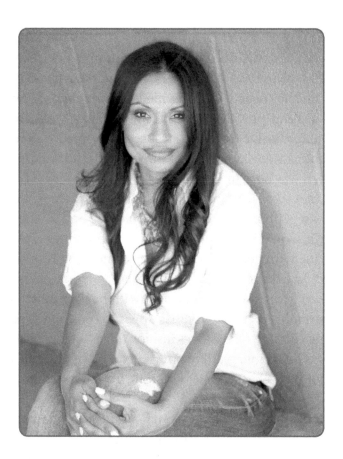